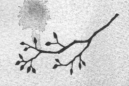

Mindful
Walking

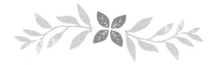

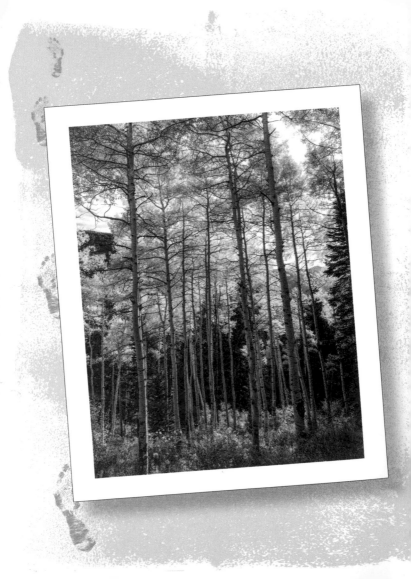

Mindful
Walking

the secret language of nature

ALICE PECK

CICO BOOKS
LONDON NEW YORK

Published in 2022 by CICO Books
An imprint of Ryland Peters & Small Ltd
20–21 Jockey's Fields   341 E 116th St
London WC1R 4BW   New York, NY 10029

www.rylandpeters.com

10 9 8 7 6 5 4 3 2 1

A CIP catalog record for this book is available from the Library of Congress
and the British Library.

ISBN: 978-1-80065-088-6

Printed in China

Editor: Rosie Fairhead
Designer: Fahema Khanam
Illustrator: Jenny McCabe

Commissioning editor: Kristine Pidkameny
Senior commissioning editor: Carmel Edmonds
Art director: Sally Powell
Head of production: Patricia Harrington
Publishing manager: Penny Craig
Publisher: Cindy Richards

FSC
MIX
Paper from
responsible sources
FSC® C106563
www.fsc.org

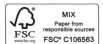
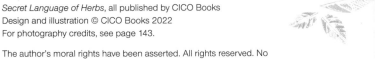

Contents

Introduction 6

Chapter 1 Take a Walk 8

Chapter 2 Forest Bathing 28

Chapter 3 Delightful Dirt 52

Chapter 4 Being in Nature 74

Chapter 5 Engaging Your Senses 90

Chapter 6 Water Treatment 108

Chapter 7 Open a Window 124

Notes 136

Photography Credits 143

Introduction

I'm optimistic by nature, and seldom morbid, but when I'm feeling low, one of my favorite places to wander is Green-Wood Cemetery in Brooklyn, New York. It is glorious and green and quiet—very quiet. When roaming its 478 acres (193 hectares) in the middle of the most populated city in the United States, I've seen warblers and water lilies, and gathered acorns and my thoughts. The verdure, the serenity, and the frogsong all bring me back to life. I am by no means the first person to have this regenerative experience. Regardless of who we are or where we live, what we all know intuitively is that going outside is good for us.

Any kind of walking is good for you, but when you walk outdoors, you will get vitamin D—the sunshine vitamin, and you will experience a better physical and mental workout navigating uneven outdoor terrain rather than pounding the consistent surface of a treadmill. Another bonus is that it is hard to be on a smartphone or other device when you are walking outside, so you will also give yourself a break from screens. Other benefits of going for a walk include being able to greet and maybe get to know other walkers, thereby connecting with people and building community, and doing your own small part for the environment by picking up a bit of trash to improve the aesthetics of your route.

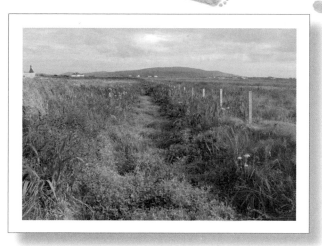

Most of all, you will feel refreshed by a walk: it's a way
to dust the cobwebs from your mind, welcome a new
perspective on the day or on life, and get the blood
flowing. Taking a walk can help your physical and mental
health—and ultimately, as you'll discover in this book,
change your life.

In every walk with nature, one
receives far more than he seeks.

John Muir in *Steep Trails* (1918)

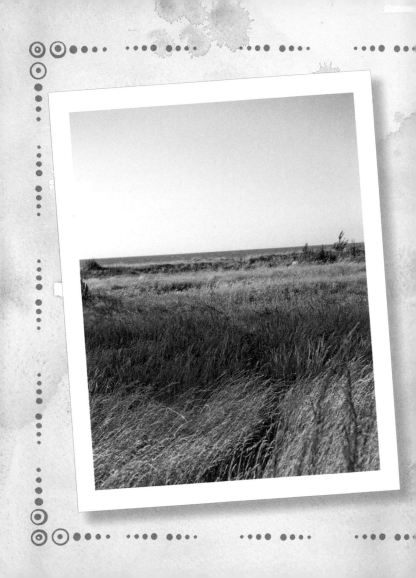

Chapter 1

Take a Walk

Change Your Life by Walking

The great thing about reaping the benefits of walking is that we don't have to do very much to change our health for the better. In most of the research I have read, 150 seems to be the magic number: People who engaged in 150 minutes of walking per week showed marked improvements and benefits to their health. So, if you can, make moving for at least 25 minutes six times a week your goal. Consider walking the dog or strolling to the market, getting off the subway or bus a stop before your destination, taking the scenic route home, running up and down the stairs in your apartment building on rainy days. All these things can change your life significantly.

Of course, the more you walk, the better, but experts say that while it's good to aim for a whole lot of steps, your focus should be on sustaining consistent daily minimums, not sporadically pushing yourself to reach a record number of steps. A sports tracking device or smartphone app could come in handy with this. It will help you to keep track of time and see how quickly 25 minutes can pass when you're both in motion and in nature.

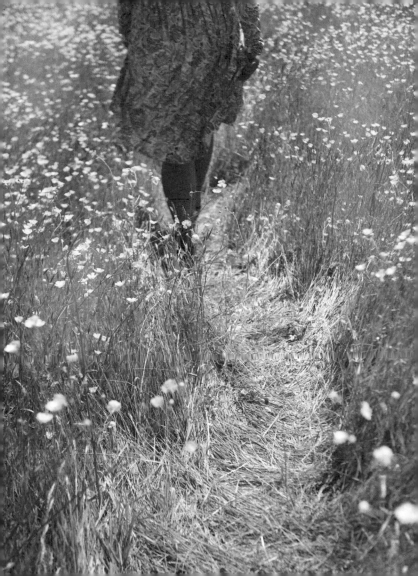

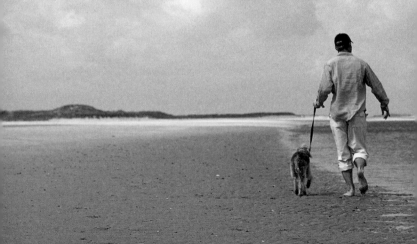

Above all, do not lose your desire to walk: Every day, I walk myself into a state of wellbeing and walk away from every illness; I have walked myself into my best thoughts, and I know of no thought so burdensome that one cannot walk away from it.

Søren Kierkegaard (1813–1855), from a letter to his sister-in-law Henriette

Stand Up

Healthcare practitioners claim that chairs are the new cigarettes. Seriously—too much sitting can kill you! Or, as Kierkegaard put it, "the more one sits still, the closer one comes to feeling ill."[1]

Research from the University of California found that sitting for too long—like smoking—increases the risk of diabetes, heart disease, and even early death. The researchers found a connection between sedentary behavior and thinning in parts of the brain that are responsible for forming memories.[2] This can be a precursor to dementia and other types of cognitive decline, and middle-aged and older adults should be especially aware of it.

A famous comprehensive study published in the *Journal of Clinical Nutrition*, analyzing 240,000 Americans between the ages of 50 and 71, showed a direct correlation between sitting and mortality.[3] The more we sit, the sooner we die. It sounds dire indeed, but the good news is that the converse is also true: By getting up and moving we delay the onset of many age-related problems.

The Benefits of Walking

The effect of aerobic and ambulatory exercise on Alzheimer's disease was studied by scientists at the University of Kansas. Half the test subjects engaged in walking and brisk movement, while the other half did toning and stretching exercises. All showed some improvement in tests for physical skills, but what is fascinating is that "some of the walkers significantly increased their scores on cognitive tests that focused on thinking and remembering. The brain's hippocampus, the area most closely linked to memory retrieval, had in some cases actually grown."[4] Think about that: We can develop our brains by taking regular walks.

Walking has an especially significant impact on the vagus, the nerve that connects our brain to our body, branching out to our primary organs (heart, lungs, and digestive tract). It's the nerve that makes the mind/body connection. When you activate the vagus nerve by walking, deep breathing, steady stretching, or doing yoga or any kind of rhythmic exercise, it regulates your adrenal gland. This gland produces hormones in stressful situations, and modulates blood pressure and the flow of blood to the organs, especially the heart, allowing them to function more efficiently and effectively.[5]

OTHER WAYS WALKING HELPS

Reduces inflammation, osteoporosis, and cardiovascular disease

Enhances balance, posture, and joint fluidity, and even lowers the incidence of vascular dementia

Improves digestive health and the functioning of the colon

Increases "good" cholesterol levels, and lowers triglycerides or "bad" cholesterol [6]

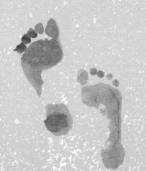

Happier in Motion

It's not just in our bodies that we see the benefits of fresh air and movement; with physical fitness comes psychological fitness. Poets, painters, scientists, and efficiency experts have all commented on how outdoor exercise in nature works as a balm for our minds and a way to de-stress. How many times have you taken a walk around the block to cool off?

Former competitive racewalker and cancer survivor Carolyn Scott Kortge supports this idea in her book *Healing Walks for Hard Times* (2010). She reveals how taking a walk is about far more than exercise; it can serve as "a form of stress release and healing that supports medical treatment and emotional recovery." The basic ambulatory act increases our exhalations and inhalations, causing us to release endorphins—from the term "endogenous morphine"—that trigger a natural opioid effect, making us feel happier and more optimistic, while decreasing our perception of pain. It's those hormones that cause the well-known "runner's high."

Numerous studies have shown that walking encourages the front region of our brain—the hypothalamus, which controls temperature, thirst, and hunger, and affects sleep and emotions—to manufacture oxytocin, often known as the love hormone. This acts as a neurotransmitter in the brain, stimulating feelings of empathy and affection. And with love often comes happiness. Walking can make us more joyful. A series of studies by the University of Michigan showed that this was true no matter one's age—from schoolchildren to the elderly.[7]

WALK AWAY WORRIES

These health benefits have to do with overriding rumination—our tendency to dwell on troubling thoughts or worry about everything from finances to our child's hurt feelings. These are the kinds of thoughts tinged with sorrow that we can't seem to let go of. Long-term rumination, marked by activity in the part of the brain that controls emotions and the personality (the prefrontal cortex), can lead to depression. Walking in nature has been shown to decrease rumination. A Stanford University study found that taking a 90-minute walk through a natural environment as opposed to an urban one reduces rumination and consequently the neural activity in the part of the brain that is linked to the risk of mental illness.[8] Findings such as these reinforce why green spaces are so crucial for good mental health, especially for those of us who live in urban areas.

When it comes to happiness, how you walk matters. According to the *Journal of Behavior Therapy and Experimental Psychiatry*, people who were instructed to

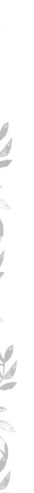

walk in a happier manner, with a lively, energetic gait, experienced more positive thoughts (as indicated by biofeedback testing, which monitors indicators like heart and breathing rate and blood pressure), recalled them more readily, and had fewer depressive tendencies.[9] It is like the expression "acting as if": If you act as if you feel better, you begin to feel (at least a little) better.

NATURE VS CITY

Myriad articles and studies detail the cognitive benefits of interacting with nature, in part because it captures our attention subtly ("Is that a bluebird?"), as opposed to walking in an urban environment ("Watch out for that car!"). This was quantified by researchers from the University of Michigan, who examined memory tests of students after sending them for a brief walk in an arboretum. They showed a 20% improvement in memory after interacting with nature, even in wintry weather, so it was the outdoors and not specifically the greenery that seemed to help.[10]

A study presented in the Proceedings of the National Academy of Sciences in 2015 supported this. Its researchers found that walking in a park reduced blood flow to a part of the brain that causes rumination, thereby improving positive focus.[11]

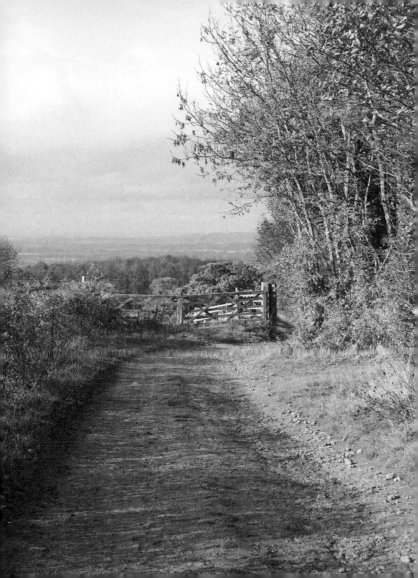

Spark Creativity

In his essay "The Etiquette of Freedom" in *The Practice of the Wild* (1990), the poet and ecologist Gary Snyder describes walking as "the great adventure, the first meditation, a practice of heartiness and soul primary to humankind ... the exact balance of spirit and humility." Recent Harvard University studies on green space and health confirm what he said: That walking heals our spirits, even our creative spirits, as well as our bodies and minds.

Writers from Henry David Thoreau to Rebecca Solnit, and Jean-Jacques Rousseau to Jane Austen, have pointed out the link between walking and creativity. Two researchers at Stanford University, Marily Oppezzo and Daniel Schwartz, analyzed this theory and found that walking—whether outdoors or indoors—enhanced creativity, especially when brainstorming new ideas. It didn't matter whether the subjects walked on a treadmill facing a bare wall or out in nature; test results showed that participants who walked before being asked to find creative solutions to problems performed twice as well as those who remained sedentary.[12]

RAMBLES, TREKS, AND WANDERINGS

Walking outdoors can be especially good for the spirit, which is perhaps why people have always been drawn to pilgrimages such as the Camino de Santiago (popularized during the Middle Ages as a route of Christian pilgrimage, the paths through northwest Spain are still a favorite among hikers of all faiths) or the trail to the Shinto shrine at the top of the Nachi Falls in Wakayama Prefecture, southern Japan. This is a way of embodying the sacred journey, as our inner, mental voyage is reflected and marked by an outer, physical one.

A trudge through a vacant lot can be as beneficial as a stroll through a meadow, if it's all that is available. Whether it is a pilgrimage or a trip around the block, try to find time each day to engage with the world around you, being present and appreciating the simple beauties of nature. Try taking off your headphones, or—and this is really hard for me, because I like a purpose, whether it is a trip to the market or exercising the dog—try ambling, walking without a purpose or destination in mind.

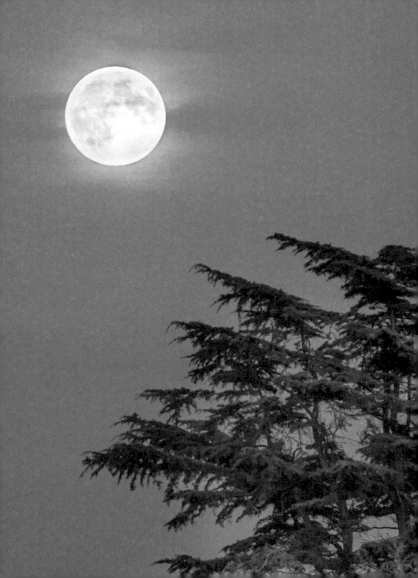

WALKING AT NIGHT

There are many reasons to recommend the writer and former Zen Buddhist monk Clark Strand's beautiful meditation on sleep, dark, and light, *Waking Up to the Dark* (2015). He writes about how our nightly patterns break into three parts when we are removed from artificial light for a significant amount of time: About four hours of deep sleep, two hours of awakened quiet rest, then four more hours of sleep. One of my favorite things about Strand's book is his descriptions of walking at night:

*"If someone asked me why I rise to walk at night,
I couldn't answer except to say that I do it for its own sake,
for the sake of rising and walking and praying in the dark.
That time of contemplation and communion is its own
reward. It creates its own culture in the soul."*[13]

Ever since I read Strand's treatise about the things we can see without artificial light, I've been taking little walks in the dark—not the mountain hikes he describes, but around my house or into the backyard in darkness. It's a kind of meditation: By removing visual distractions we can become more present and more mindful of where we are.

Walking Meditation

The Vietnamese Buddhist teacher and peace activist Thich Nhat Hanh wrote in *Present Moment, Wonderful Moment* (1990):

"The mind can go in a thousand directions. But on this beautiful path, I walk in peace. With each step, a gentle wind blows. With each step, a flower blooms."[14]

Like exercise, the benefits of meditation are many, and scientists and doctors are always finding new ones, from easing stress to improving focus to facilitating healing on all levels from heart health to immunity. There is a way to combine both exercise and meditation, and you can do it outside in nature, whether that nature is a sylvan glade, a seashore path, or the sidewalk between apartment buildings.

Here is a walking meditation practice based on the zen technique *kinhin*, which might seem familiar if you have ever intentionally walked a labyrinth. It can be done inside or outdoors, but try for as much fresh air and greenery as possible. It's best to plan your route in advance. Knowing your destination means you won't have to make decisions and can pay attention to each step.

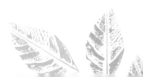

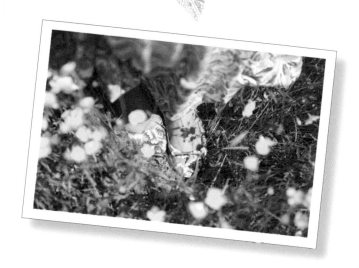

1 Stand up straight and take a deep breath.

••••⊙⊙⊙••••

2 Hold your hands in such a way that they don't swing
around but won't cramp either. I like to fold mine in
front of me, the left held in the right.

••••⊙⊙⊙••••

3 Synchronize your breath with your pace. Inhale and step slowly and deliberately, exhale and take another step.

••••◉◎◉•••

4 Begin to walk, paying attention to lifting your foot and placing it on the ground, then lifting your other foot and placing it on the ground.

••••◉◎◉•••

5 Continue to walk in this careful, controlled manner. Don't force it, but don't saunter either.

••••◉◎◉•••

6 As with any mindfulness practice, when thoughts arise, look at them and let them go. Don't ignore, don't judge.

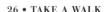

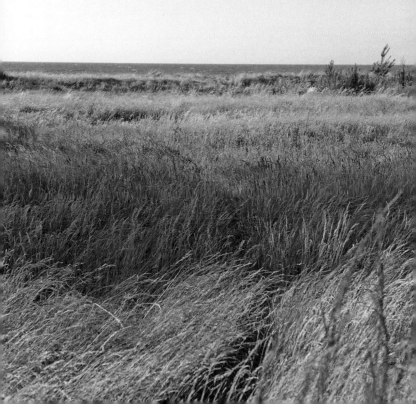

Breathing in, I know Mother Earth is in me.
Breathing out, I know Mother Earth is in me.

Thich Nhat Hanh (1926–)

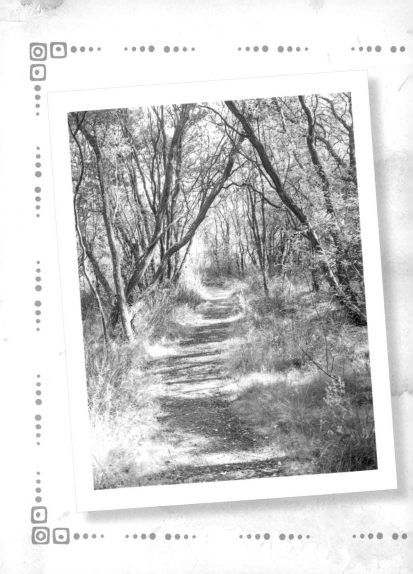

Chapter 2

Forest Bathing

A Love of Trees

Any walk outdoors is good for you, but if you can get to some woods, that's even better. Over the past few years, more people have become intrigued by the concept of forest bathing—healing through the contemplative practice of intentionally spending time with trees.

As humans, we are drawn to trees. It's an innate tendency that transcends borders and cultures, and something powerful happens to us when we are near them. People often respond with delight to a mention of trees, and many will describe a tree that's special to them. In his wildly popular book *Forest Bathing: How Trees Can Help You Find Health and Happiness* (2018), Dr. Qing Li explains that there is a Japanese word for that indescribable feeling: *yūgen*, meaning "deep" and "mysterious." In the Japanese system of aesthetics, it is understood as a profound and sometimes poignant wonder at the beauty of the universe.

Yūgen is one of many reasons that forest bathing has caught on, but there are more: It is a lovely way to pass the time in nature and it enables us to connect to the spiritual without dogma.

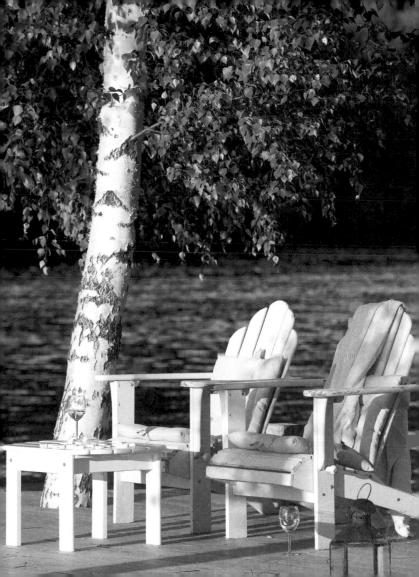

The Health Benefits
of Trees

In 1982, Tomohide Akiyama, then secretary of Japan's Ministry of Agriculture, Forestry, and Fisheries, coined the term shinrin-yoku. This translates as "forest bathing," and can be defined as making contact with and being affected—both physically and mentally—by the atmosphere of the forest. Perhaps more aptly called forest basking, since neither soap nor tub is involved, forest bathing can be experienced as a type of meditation, and, just as with other Eastern-rooted practices such as mindfulness, Ayurvedic medicine, and yoga, Westerners are learning that there is far more to meditation than simply becoming calm. Many authorities are in agreement that meditation can ease psychological problems from anxiety to post-traumatic stress disorder, help to treat addiction, make us better parents and workers, and promote the healing of many physical ailments.

Forest bathing incorporates many of the benefits of meditation while getting us outdoors and in motion. In a recent study conducted by the College of Landscape Architecture at Sichuan Agricultural University, Chengdu,

China, 30 men and 30 women were given a route of the same length to walk in either a bamboo forest or an urban area. The results showed that, although walking is good for you, walking among trees is much better.[1] The researchers measured blood pressure as well as electrical activity in the brain using an EEG (electroencephalogram), and they found that, among those who walked the forest path, blood pressure was lowered significantly as attention and concentration improved. The people walking in nature reported less anxiety and a generally happier mood than the urban group.

I frequently tramped eight or ten miles through the deepest snow to keep an appointment with a beech-tree, or a yellow birch, or an old acquaintance among the pines.

Henry David Thoreau, *Walden* (1854)

FURTHER BENEFITS OF FOREST BATHING

Forest bathing has an impact on even more than mood and blood pressure. The New York State Department of Environmental Conservation and myriad other sources maintain that the simple act of intentional, attentive time with trees:

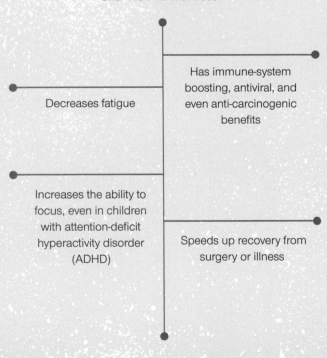

Has immune-system boosting, antiviral, and even anti-carcinogenic benefits

Decreases fatigue

Increases the ability to focus, even in children with attention-deficit hyperactivity disorder (ADHD)

Speeds up recovery from surgery or illness

Increases energy

Lowers blood glucose,
affecting obesity
and diabetes

Regulates the endocrine
(hormonal) system

Has been shown to increase
brainwave activity in young
adults and improve the health
of elderly patients with
chronic heart failure [2]

Enhances the ability to
relax and get a better
night's sleep

Phytoncides

Forest bathing is an active process, not just a matter of being near trees as static objects. Many species, including pine, yew, hop hornbeam, and sugi, emit biochemicals called phytoncides that interact with our central nervous system and have calming, anesthetic qualities, even anti-carcinogenic properties. Phytoncides are pungent essential oils and antimicrobial volatile organic compounds. When you are breathing in the heady fragrance of pine or cedar, you are inhaling phytoncides. They have been proven to boost the trees' health as well as our immune systems, which is a powerful thing, but that's not the only benefit of forest bathing.

Phytoncides contain terpenes (like those in cannabidiol, CBD, a chemical compound found in marijuana oil) that can stimulate immunity and anti-cancer proteins in our bodies, fight viruses, and increase the release of the steroid hormone dehydroepiandrosterone (DHEA) into the blood, protecting and even strengthening our hearts. They also activate the vagus nerve (see page 14), reduce our production of the stress hormone cortisol[3] (making us more calm and focused), and likely decrease inflammation, as well.

FINDING THE RIGHT TREES

It is important to note that not all forests are rich in phytoncides. German forester and writer Peter Wohlleben points out in *The Hidden Life of Trees* (2015) that when spruce and pine trees are introduced to places where they're not indigenous, the trees suffer, dry out, and create excess dust, making us less, not more, healthy, so be aware when seeking out a forest to walk in or planting trees.

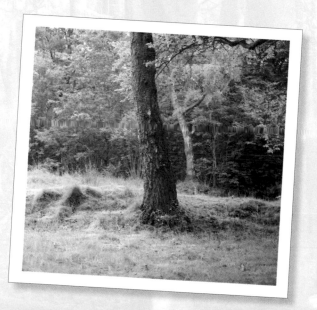

Natural Air Purifiers

As trees emit, they also absorb. According to Wohlleben, trees act as natural air purifiers, not unlike houseplants. Trees take in pollutants such as nitrogen oxide, ammonia, sulfur dioxide, and ozone through their leaves. That's part of why we feel better when we go for a walk in the woods. Breathing cleaner air is not just a pleasant experience; it can reduce the symptoms of asthma, make exercise more efficient because we don't have to work as hard to take in oxygen, and perhaps even mildly cleanse our organs.

In the woods, we return to reason and faith. There I feel that nothing can befall me in life—no disgrace, no calamity ... which nature cannot repair. Standing on the bare ground, my head bathed by the blithe air, and uplifted into infinite space ... the currents of the Universal Being circulate through me.

Ralph Waldo Emerson, *Nature* (1836)

Fractals

Fractals are structures in which the same pattern recurs at a progressively smaller scale. Think about how the vein patterns of a leaf echo the appearance of the tree itself. The geometry of fractals is all around us—zoom in on a fern, a pine tree, a snowflake, a snail shell, a Queen Anne's lace flower, or a head of broccoli, and you'll find fractals. Dr. Qing Li (see page 30) incorporates them into his forest bathing instructions, and writes that after gazing at fractals, first as light through a tree canopy and then as leaves, parts of leaves, and veins, we can appreciate the interconnected patterns of the natural world. With that appreciation can come sensations of wonder and delight, as well as of quietude and tranquility.[4]

Richard Taylor, professor of physics at the University of Oregon, is developing retinal implants to restore vision for people suffering from eye disease. In the process he looked at images of Jackson Pollock's action paintings. At first you might think this is a stretch—from Abstract Expressionist painting to inner eye implants—but it was through Pollock's art that Taylor first realized how nature's fractals might relate to human stress. Because of this, he made sure that the implants he developed simulated the retina's design to induce the same kind of stress reduction that would result when looking at nature's fractals through healthy eyes.

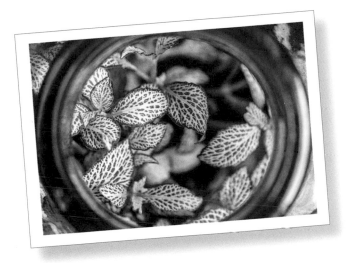

Taylor found that seeing fractals stimulates the pleasure centers in the brain, but it went further than that. When his team used EEGs to monitor electrical activity in the brain and electrical responses in the skin of their subjects, they found that looking at works of art—such as Pollock's paintings— produced a reduction in stress of 60%. That's with no medication, no mantras, no stretches or yoga poses, just looking at a fractal-rich painting. They also discovered that the physiological change initiated by looking at the art accelerated recovery from surgery.[5] Mind-blowing!

Hearing Trees

It has been scientifically proven that trees emit not just an aerosol of healing phytoncides, but also beneficial sounds. We've all heard branches groan in a storm and the susurration or whispering of leaves as they move together in an afternoon breeze, but plants (and trees in particular) also emit vibrations that can be measured using microphones and ultrasonic sensors. In an interview with *Yale Environment 360* in 2017, the biologist David George Haskell explained that "an ultrasonic detector applied to a tree, particularly in the summertime, reveals how as the morning passes into afternoon, the tree goes from a state of full hydration to a place of distress, where there are all sorts of little ultrasonic clicks and fizzles emerging from the inside of the tree as water columns break, as the tree becomes more dried out."[6]

Just as trees respond to increases and decreases in light and temperature, they also respond to sound via vibrations. For example, urban trees tend to grow thicker bark as a reaction to the shaking and pulsation of passing traffic. There are also hypotheses that trees use sounds to communicate with one another. In an interview in *Smithsonian* magazine, Wohlleben calls this the "wood-wide web": The connection among trees in a healthy forest, whereby nutrients and water are shared and information sent by means of a symbiotic relationship underground, between microscopic filaments at the tips of tree roots and fungi—called mycorrhizal networks—to signal threats such as drought or insect infestation.[7]

If trees can emit vibrations, it follows that human beings can pick them up, even if only on a very subtle level. I spoke to several proponents of forest bathing who say that those vibrations can cure headaches more quickly and naturally than taking an analgesic. I haven't had that experience, but when my thoughts are unsettled, if I sit with the silver maple in my backyard I feel better. Is it the vibrations, the terpenes, the green of the leaves, or the pause to reflect on something that has endured more than a hundred years of blizzards, thunderstorms, and heatwaves? I'm not sure, but I know it heals me in a unique way.

QUIVERING LEAVES

As a child, I was fascinated by aspen trees and how animated their leaves appeared. In summer, I would look to them to gauge the weather, since I knew the saying, "When leaves show their undersides, be very sure rain betides." You will appreciate the truth in this if you observe aspen leaves fluttering as they react to the increase in humidity preceding a storm. There is so much motion because their petioles, the leafstalks that join the leaves, are long and flattened and tremble, or quake, in the slightest breeze. This is why we think of aspens as whispering, tremulous, and even magical.

Now that I'm older, I'm more intrigued that a tree can represent communication, and for me the aspen helps to put life into perspective and demonstrates how to acknowledge the interconnection of all beings. Aspens are surculose, having long root suckers that travel laterally, some as far as 26 ft (8 m) from the original tree trunk. They grow in clonal—genetically identical—colonies, derived from a single seedling. Some of these root colonies live for thousands of years, perhaps as long as 80,000 years.

One of the oldest living colonies of quaking aspens is the Pando (which means "I spread" in Latin) in Fishlake National Forest, Utah. Nicknamed the "Trembling Giant," these 105 acres (42 hectares) of aspens are connected by a single root system. The trees die off, but new shoots continue to spring up. Aspens even survive forest fires: Although the leaves, branches, and trunks above ground may be burned, the tenacious roots endure, sending up new shoots in the spring. There is poetry to a colony of trees being one of the oldest living organisms on Earth yet still producing new growth at this very moment.

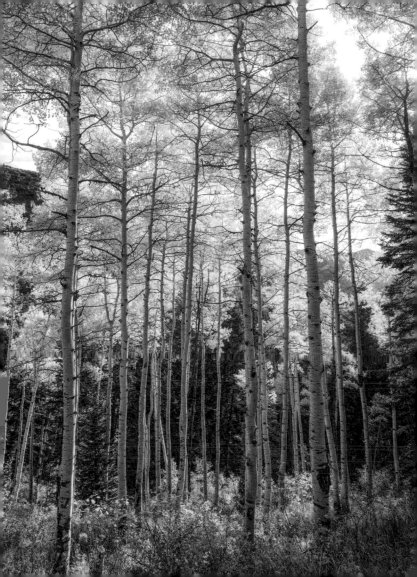

City Trees

We can't all get to the woods, but fortunately, as we've already seen, there are health benefits to even a little bit of nature. A park, a tree-lined road, or a couple of trees in a backyard or courtyard can help.

Urban planners and environmental scientists are taking the benefits of forest bathing to heart and working to create more effective green spaces. One initiative is City Tree, which isn't a tree at all, but rather a structure built from mosses that bind with toxins and particulates to clean the air.[8] It looks a bit like a giant television, but instead of a flat screen, a huge patch of moss covers the vertical surface. Not only does the moss clean the air, but also, because it stores a considerable amount of moisture, it cools the area around it.

Projects to plant (real) city trees are cropping up all over the world as urban planners learn more and more about the power of green. The MillionTreesNYC initiative was launched by the New York City Parks Department in 2007, and the project's goal was achieved in 2015. A million street trees were planted throughout the city over a period of eight years. As part of the scheme, the non-profit New York Restoration Project targeted neighborhoods that needed trees, and sought out public and private funding to provide them. Other cities, including London, Shanghai, Denver, and Los Angeles, have developed similar programs, and the results are all good—cheering up neighborhoods, raising property values, filtering air, and decreasing noise pollution.

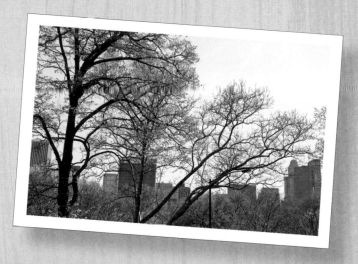

Step by Step, Tree by Tree

So, how do you go about forest bathing?

1 You need only the most basic equipment: Walking shoes and insect repellent. Leave your camera, journal, and guidebooks behind, and turn off your mobile devices. Forest bathing is about being, not analyzing.

2 Find some trees. This can be a forest of ancient pine or a copse of paper birch, or, if you're like me, a single silver maple in your backyard. Of course, spending more time with more trees is better, because the effect is multiplied—studies have shown that spending three days and two nights in a thickly wooded area will improve the function of the immune system for up to seven days—but do the best you can. A little forest bathing is better than none.

3 Find somewhere to sit or lean, where you can be still for 10 or 20 minutes or more without being in the way of bicycle traffic, ants, or poison ivy.

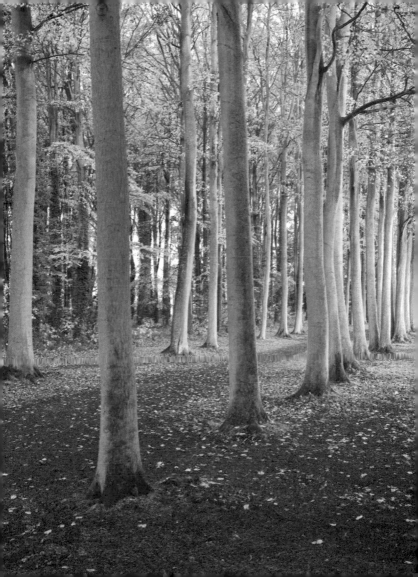

4 Now just be still. Be aware of your breath, but do not force it. Let the experience come to you, don't analyze. See what you see, hear what you hear, smell what you smell, feel what you feel. Light through the leaves ... skittering or birdsong ... blossom or decay ... calm or grounded ...

5 As you walk home, check in with yourself. Do you notice any changes in your body? How about your state of mind? What can you take back to your daily life from your forest bathing experience? Do you feel more optimistic? More serene? How is that headache?

6 Repeat as often as possible, and pay attention to any improvement in your wellbeing. Try a new spot next time, or focus on another kind of tree, and note the difference. (Having said that, forest bathing with the same trees in the same spot will vary every time, depending on the season, the weather, the time of day, and what you bring to the experience.)

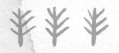

TREES IN PERPETUITY

If you're hoping your great-grandchildren will have clean
air to breathe, tend a tree! Make sure it is watered, pick
up any trash nearby, perhaps build a little fence around
it to protect it from dogs. As you do so, you could recite
this passage from the Mohawk version of the
Thanksgiving Address:

*"We now turn our thoughts to the Trees. The Earth has
many families of Trees who have their own instructions
and uses. Some provide us with shelter and shade, others
with fruit, beauty, and other useful things.*

*Many people of the world use a Tree as a symbol
of peace and strength. With one mind, we greet and
thank the Tree life. Now our minds are one."*

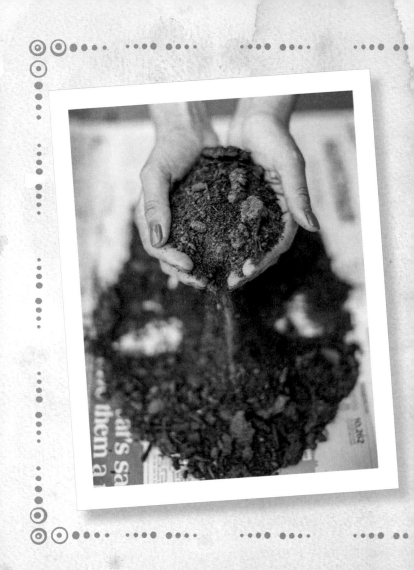

Chapter 3

Delightful Dirt

Earthing

Consider the fragrant and beautiful lotus flower—a symbol of divine perfection, especially for Hindus and Buddhists. It grows best in the mud. As the Vietnamese spiritual teacher Thich Nhat Hanh often says, "No mud, no lotus." Although our culture tends to shun dirt—and often for good reason—maybe we have gone too far. A bit of mud can be a wonderful thing. Toddlers who find joy in splashy, squishy springtime mud puddles may be onto something.

Accordingly, the earthing movement is catching on. (Some say it's the next forest bathing!) Earthing involves walking barefoot and connecting directly to the soil without the barrier of pavement or shoes. It is a matter of making contact with our soil, our planet, of truly touching the earth. More a question of appreciation than a scientific concept, earthing is also a way of connecting to others and celebrating nature.

Some people take the idea a step farther, reaching beyond the biological material to the electromagnetic charge generated by our planet. The science is still fairly new and limited on this subject, but interesting nonetheless. According to the *Journal of Inflammation Research*, wide-ranging studies have shown how the

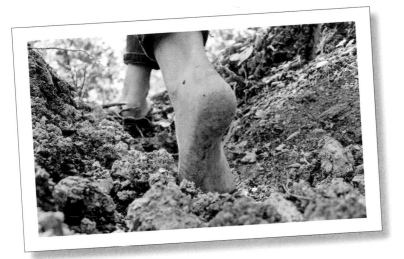

electrically conductive contact between human bodies and the Earth's surface—known as grounding (or earthing)—seems to have a positive effect on health. Sparking this connection between people and the ground we walk on may diminish inflammation, enhance immunity and wound healing, and prevent or even treat chronic inflammatory and autoimmune diseases. Grounding may also lessen pain by altering the numbers of circulating white blood cells (neutrophils and lymphocytes) affecting inflammation.[1] It sounds promising and will certainly bear more research.

Think of the non-scientific meaning of the word "grounded"—balanced, sensible, understanding what's important in life—and it follows that standing firmly on the earth, bonded to where we came from and where we'll end up, will have an impact.

TAKING ROOT IN THE MUD

In Sanskrit, the banyan is called the "tree of many feet" because of the way its many roots spread. There are several famous banyan trees, especially in India. One in particular, on a bank of India's Nerbudda River and reputedly planted by the 15th-century poet and saint Kabir, was long believed to be the oldest in the country, until it was destroyed by a flood. Another spectacular example is Thimmamma Marrimanu (*marri* means "banyan," and *manu* "tree" in Telugu) in the Indian state of Andhra Pradesh. According to *Guinness World Records*, it is the world's biggest banyan, with branches spreading over 5 acres (2 hectares), and a canopy of almost 23,000 square yards (21,000 sq m). It's so vast that a small Hindu temple has been built within its massive trunk. The banyan, which is sacred in Hinduism, is often depicted with the god Shiva sitting under its canopy, and saints gathered at his feet.

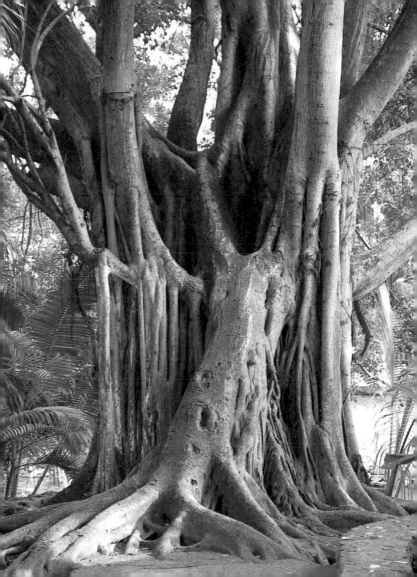

Mentioned in books by many 19th-century naturalists, the banyan has continued to inspire in recent times. Mahatma Gandhi created the term *Satyagraha*, loosely translated as "polite insistence on the truth." He wrote in 1919: "Satyagraha is like a banyan tree ... *Satya* (truth) and *ahimsa* (non-violence) together make the present trunk from which innumerable branches shoot out ... We must fearlessly spread the doctrine of *satya* and *ahimsa*, and then, and not till then, shall we be able to undertake mass *satyagraha*." This form of non-violent resistance influenced many, including Martin Luther King, Jr., during the American Civil Rights Movement, and Nelson Mandela in his struggle against apartheid in South Africa.

'Tis not in the high stars alone,
Nor in the cup of budding flowers,
Nor in the redbreast's mellow tone,
Nor in the bow that smiles in showers,
But in the mud and scum of things
There alway, alway something sings.

Ralph Waldo Emerson, from "Music" in *Poems* (1904)

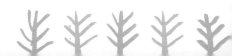

Ground Yourself

Like the non-violent protester, the banyan will not be moved. It is grounded and fixed to the earth by a multitude of connections. Be like the banyan by trying the tree pose from yoga. Begin by standing, concentrating on feeling grounded with your gaze fixed forward. Now lift a foot and place it on the opposite thigh. Bring your hands together on your chest as if in prayer and consider the banyan tree soaring upward yet always rooted.

Mud Baths

If walking barefoot isn't your thing, consider fangotherapy—a mud bath! Studies have shown that applying mud to the skin can relieve psoriasis and atopic dermatitis as well as rosacea, eczema, acne, and generally itchy skin. Fangotherapy has also had proven results in treating neurological, rheumatologic (osteoarthritis), and even some cardiovascular disorders.[2] Researchers at the Kaplan Medical Center in Rehovot, Israel, found that using mudpacks and mineral-water soaks to absorb minerals through the skin may benefit our immune system. For example, sulfur baths have been successfully used to treat types of dermatitis and psoriasis, and have shown potential in regulating the skin's immune response as a treatment for allergic reactions.[3]

Where the mud comes from determines its benefits. It's those microbes again! The scientists at the Kaplan Medical Center analyzed mud from the Dead Sea, which is especially rich in organic substances such as calcium, magnesium, and potassium, and not the mud you might dredge up from the bottom of your local lake, for example. The makeup of the mud not only allows nutrients to be absorbed into the skin, but also means that it retains heat for a long time, stimulating blood flow—nature's heating pad.

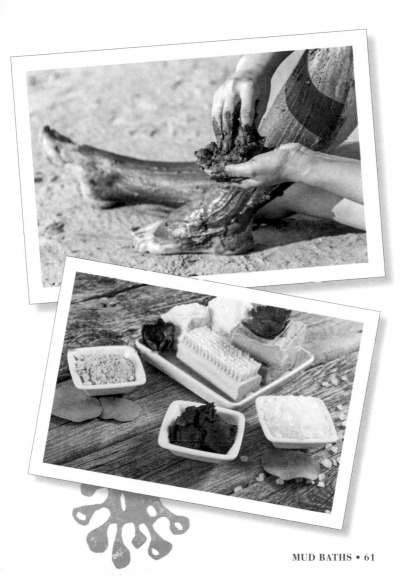

Mud Medicine

Anyone who gardens knows that digging in the earth makes them feel better, and now there's science to back it up. "Good" bacteria form part of microbiomes that build our resistance to illness and fight the "bad" bacteria that cause infection. These microbiomes reside in specific environments, such as our gut, our skin, and the soil.

In 2004, after learning about the successful results of using bacteria to treat drug-resistant pulmonary tuberculosis, a British oncologist injected the microorganism Mycobacterium vaccae (SRL172) into patients with non-small-cell lung cancer to see if it would strengthen their immune systems. It didn't work, but there was a different and surprising result: When SRL172 was combined with chemotherapy, it significantly improved the quality of the patients' lives.[4] As indicated by their global health score (a standardized measure of respondents' evaluation of their health), those who received the injections of bacteria were happier and livelier, and had improved cognitive function.

In part because of this, three American and international research groups—the University of Chicago, the Marine Biological Laboratory, and Argonne National Laboratory— have joined together to form the Microbiome Center,

a coordinated interdisciplinary research group. Its director, Jack Gilbert, explains that the microbes in our guts communicate with our brains in several ways.[5] They activate the immune system and produce neurotransmitters (chemical messengers between nerve cells), including 90% of our serotonin. This is important because serotonin contributes to happiness and wellbeing. Targeted treatments using the microbiome show promise in treating people suffering from PTSD and depression.

All this research boils down to something quite simple: Encourage your children to play in the mud! According to the pediatric neurologist Maya Shetreat-Klein MD, author of *The Dirt Cure* (2016), when we kill "bad" bugs—whether insects or germs—by over- or misusing pesticides, antibiotics, and hand sanitizers, we're also killing the good" bugs that prevent ailments such as asthma, allergies, eczema, and other autoimmune problems.

To nurture a garden is to feed not just the body, but the soul.

Alfred Austin (1835–1913)

MINIMUM DAILY DIRT REQUIREMENT

How can we go about getting just the right amount of dirt? There are plenty of simple ways to meet your MDDR—minimum daily dirt requirement. Start by considering where your food comes from. Eat fruit and vegetables that have been organically grown as close as possible to where you live. You'll certainly consume fewer pesticides, and probably a little more healthy dirt, since local, farm-grown food tends to be less sterilized and scrubbed than factory varieties. (Pregnant women and anyone with a compromised immune system should always wash food thoroughly to remove soil-borne toxoplasmosis.)

When it comes to small children, it may be a simple matter of encouraging them to dig in the dirt and sit on the grass, if you have access to a bit of lawn or some flowerpots. Little ones love observing bugs and small creatures, and organizing activities or adventures around such basic interests will not only get them in contact with dirt, but also give them a break from television and small screens. As children get older, encourage outdoor sports, hiking, camping, or helping in the garden. Ask your school what programs they provide to get kids outdoors—perhaps fossil-hunting for a geology curriculum or taking local soil samples for biology study.

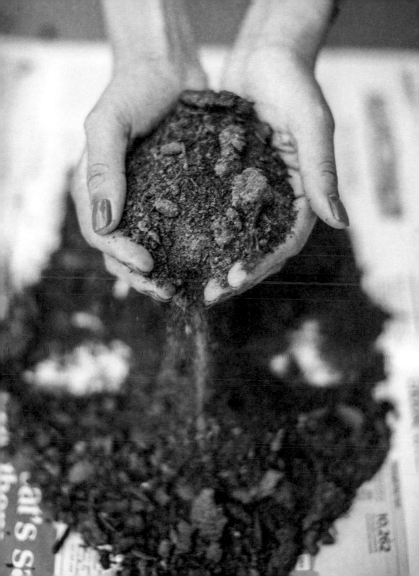

Eat Dirt?

Of course, the beneficial effects of healthy gut bacteria aren't limited to children. Eat dirt—if that's your thing! It's called geophagy, which the dictionary defines as "the practice of eating earthy substances (such as clay) that in humans is performed especially to augment a scanty or mineral-deficient diet or as part of a cultural tradition."

It's not completely crazy. Many sources explain that the reason animals and people eat soil, which is after all organic material—the stuff of plants and animals, or a salad and steak in a different form—is to ingest minerals such as iron and calcium that are necessary for our dietary health. The nutritional anthropologist Sera Young expands on this by explaining that clay works as a type of purifying filtration system, and that "it is often used to clean up massive oil spills and absorb unwanted scents from places (think kitty litter) ... it may have a similar effect in the human body, acting as a mud mask for the gut."[6]

Young isn't talking about the clay you might dig up in your backyard, but rather about the chalky clay kaolin, from the mineral kaolinite, which is common all over the world, and eaten as a folk remedy in the American South. The science is still pretty sketchy, and the process unappealing, so I'm not going to take up geophagy at this point in my life.

A GOOD GUT DIET

Fortunately, there are other, more pleasant ways than geophagy to contribute to a good gut microbiome and get a modest amount of dirt into our systems. One way is to eat a variety of foods. Here are a few particularly beneficial options:

A plant-based diet of fruits, vegetables, and legumes—stuff that grows in the dirt. Potatoes, beets, leeks, onions, and garlic are particularly suitable. (Potatoes eaten with the peel contain about twice as much potassium as bananas, and are rich in magnesium, among other nutrients.)[7]

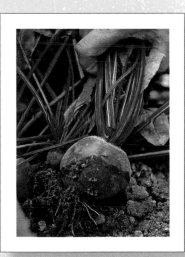

Deep-colored foods such as cocoa and blueberries that are rich in polyphenols, plant compounds that reduce blood pressure, inflammation, and cholesterol. Polyphenols aren't always absorbed efficiently or quickly by human cells, so they must work their way down to the colon, where they can "feed" or be digested by good bacteria.[8]

Prebiotic foods—foods that are high in fiber, such as wholegrains—that require other bacteria, such as Bifidobacterium, to break them down, lowering the risk of obesity, heart disease, and diabetes.[9]

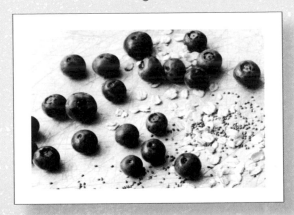

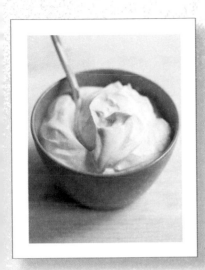

Fermented foods such as yogurt and kimchi, which contain Lactobacillus, bacteria that contribute to gut health and may even fight inflammation.[10]

Alcohol, antibiotics, smoking, and stress all have a negative impact on our gut bacteria, so limit or avoid as appropriate.

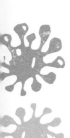

Cleansing with Mud

A trip to the Dead Sea or even to a spa in Calistoga, California, where a mud bath costs upward of $100, isn't a possibility for most of us. However, we can replicate some of the results at home.

Note: Remember that because mud is all about bacteria, you shouldn't put it on an open wound or use it with newborns or the immune suppressed.

1 Make some mud. Don't even think about dipping into your flowerpots—"clean" dirt is key. Bentonite clay or Fuller's earth (both inexpensive and available online or from health-food stores) are the best bet.

2 Mix it with water until it reaches a workable muddy consistency, not soupy but not powdery either. I use filtered or distilled water because to my mind it seems purer, but in truth, tap water is likely fine.

3 Use the mud to make a face mask. Before applying to your face, test it on a small patch of skin (such as on your arm) for about 10 minutes and wait for an hour or two to make sure you don't have any sensitivities.

Simply apply a thin paste of the mud, let it soak in and dry thoroughly for about 20 minutes, wash off completely, and moisturize as much as you need to. (Don't forget to clean the sink!) You will find that your skin looks cleaner because the mud has bonded with and absorbed oils, and that it has a bit of a glow, because when you removed the mud, it took dead skin cells with it.

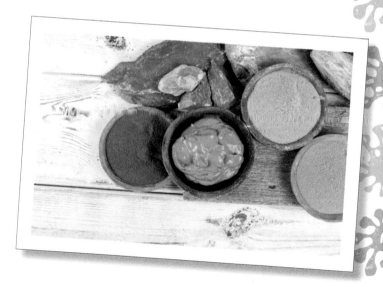

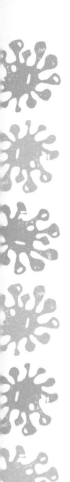

4 This is my favorite part: Get your hands dirty! I like to coat my hands with the mud mixture and let it dry. Like everyone, I use my hands constantly for everything from typing to cooking, and the mud soak feels therapeutic, warm, and toning, especially if I take the time to sit in the sun while it's drying. Once the mud has dried fully, rinse and scrub it off. This makes my hands feel remarkably clean and look a little younger, and hopefully I've absorbed some minerals in the process.

Mud can be applied to injuries, such as a sprained wrist or an arthritic knee. Although the term "mud pack" is commonly used, what is really meant is a thick mask—a heavy application of mud that is allowed to dry over the affected area. Again, heat will help, and the line between taking the time to attend to the muscle and the powers of mud itself is a blurry one.

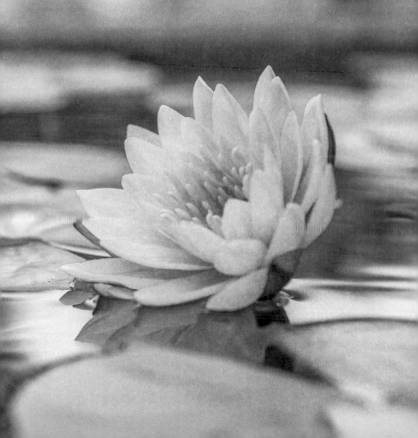

May we exist in muddy water
with purity like a lotus.

Zen Buddhist chant

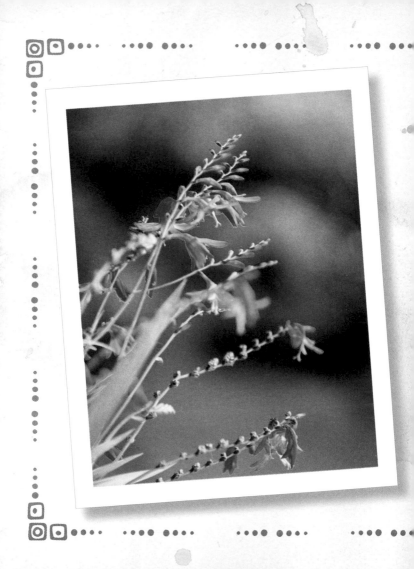

Chapter 4

Being in Nature

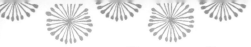

Open Spaces

The brain responds positively to open space—meadows of wildflowers, deserts that (at least from a distance) seem empty of everything but sand and light—and that can be metaphorical as well as literal. Think of the potential and excitement of a fresh notebook or a blank canvas. We've all experienced the rewards of a simple pause, a rest from stimulation. Despite what we might have been told as children, staring into "empty" space and daydreaming might in fact be time well spent.

In her lovely book *Zen of the Plains: Experiencing Wild Western Places* (2014), Tyra A. Olstad writes an ode to "windswept ridges and wind-rent skies." She describes our tendency to dismiss wide-open spaces as empty, meaningless, and blank—devoid of the complexity of ocean or woods, for example. Setting out to understand these easily overlooked areas and to learn the power of their open-ended potential, she found meaning in the "simple sweep of the horizon; the rich color of the air." She concludes the book with "a brief meditation on expectation and emptiness," picturing a snowfall: "Then there is space ... Not emptiness, nor a lack of things, much less a memory of what was once there and desire for what could be. No, in that space, there's a rich possibility, an anything, an everything."[1]

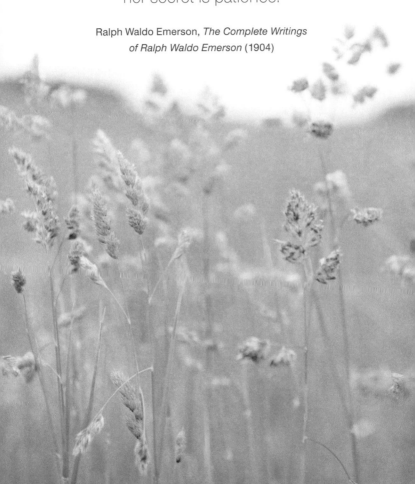

Adopt the pace of Nature;
her secret is patience.

Ralph Waldo Emerson, *The Complete Writings
of Ralph Waldo Emerson* (1904)

WILDFLOWER OF
THE MEADOW

Some call it meadow queen, or lady of the meadow. Its scent is indeed sweet, a mixture of almond and vanilla, and it makes for a wonderful potpourri. Meadowsweet is beloved by bees and sweetens their honey. Sacred to the Druids, it was used to flavor mead—a fruit and honey beverage—in the Middle Ages.

Meadowsweet's remarkably fragrant and beautiful ivory-colored blossoms are the source of its restorative qualities. Flourishing in meadows, marshes, and the moist banks of streams and ponds through most of North America, this relative of roses, almonds, and apples is sometimes called bridewort because it was strewn at weddings and crushed underfoot to release its scent.

In Italian, there is a phrase "*la dolce far niente*," which means the sweetness of doing nothing, and it is one I think suits meadowsweet. Although there are some herbalists who suggest it as a traditional treatment for soothing colds and nausea, and it does contain salicylic acid like aspirin, meadowsweet doesn't have much therapeutic or beneficial value compared to some other herbs.

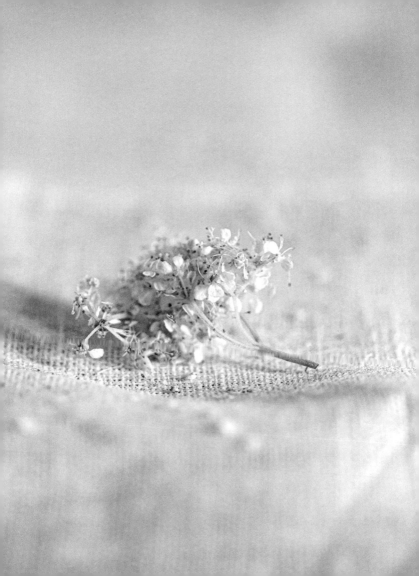

The Air Outdoors

Camping is one of the least expensive ways of taking a vacation, and has become more popular recently, perhaps in part because it allows us to escape from our digital lifestyles. However, camping is more than a craze. Some researchers consider it the best treatment for TILT (toxicant-induced loss of tolerance), a condition wherein our immune system sustains too much exposure to toxins, whether human-made pollutants such as pesticides and cleaning agents, or natural ones such as smoke, pollen, or dust mites.[2]

Getting outside every day, rather than just for camping vacations, is a key part of Scandinavian culture, known as *friluftsliv*. The term, which means "open-air living" or "free air life," was coined by the 19th-century Norwegian writer Henrik Ibsen in his poem "On the Heights," which is in part about the benefits of solitary retreat:

> *"In the lonely mountain farm,*
> *My abundant catch I take.*
> *There is a hearth, and table,*
> *And friluftsliv for my thoughts."*[3]

There is a possibility that for Ibsen, *friluftsliv* was a way to mitigate his chronic depression and anxiety. Data that compares the health of Scandinavian cultures, for whom *friluftsliv* and a connection to nature is a way of life, with that of countries or populations that neglect to spend time outdoors regularly supports this.

The benefits of fresh air go beyond easing depression. According to the Natural Resources Institute Finland and others, there is a correlation between lowered stress and a few moments of connection with green space.[4] If we spend five hours in nature outside an urban environment, preferably in two or three "doses," our mood and state of mind will improve markedly.[5] Five hours per month—less than 90 minutes a week—spending time in a park or a garden seems quite manageable for most of us.

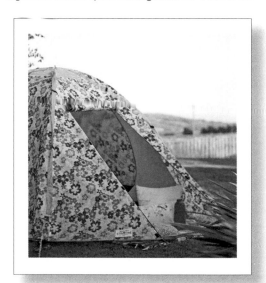

OUTSIDE IN THE CITY

We can't all get to a farm or meadow, but even spending time in limited urban green space can have a positive effect. City-dwellers breathe in a lot of polluted air from cars and industry, filled with heavy metals such as arsenic and lead, and it creates inflammation, which harms the lungs and heart. Studies have shown that we can counter this and improve our lung tissue with a walk someplace green—a nearby park, your own backyard, the courtyard of your apartment complex, or a cul-de-sac ...

Being in a meadow, field, or any other open space brings many benefits, even if it's only perceived as an open space. The Construction Industry Research and Information Association (CIRIA), an advocate for green spaces in urban settings, has found that views of or access to green spaces can improve and hasten recovery from illness or surgery and lessen the need for medication. CIRIA goes on to say that research has shown that people who live near open spaces with some element of green "seem to be more effective in managing major life issues, coping with poverty, and performing better in cognitive tasks."[6]

Even walking through the city to a park or green area has been shown to calm our minds. In 2017, using EEGs, self-reported measures, and interviews, researchers at the universities of York and Edinburgh showed that, among the elderly, "Walking between busy urban environments and green spaces triggers changes in levels of excitement, engagement, and frustration in the brain."[7]

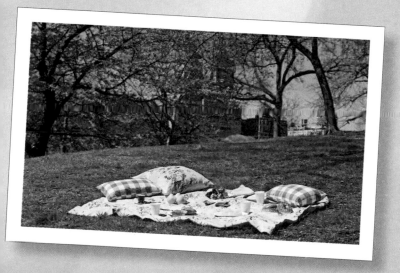

Foraging

For those of us who do have access to the countryside, there is another kind of healing to be found where things grow wild. As Robin Wall Kimmerer wrote in *Braiding Sweetgrass: Indigenous Wisdom, Scientific Knowledge, and the Teachings of Plants* (2014), "Plants know how to make food and medicine from light and water, and then they give it away."[8]

Foraging—not just in rural areas, but even in city parks—is becoming more and more popular, and offers a way to be somewhere green and find some food for "free." Berries are a great example. According to the Irish botanist and medical biochemist (and personal hero of mine!) Diana Beresford-Kroeger, wild lingonberries, blackberries, elderberries, cloudberries, raspberries, and other small fruit carry "an extraordinary biochemical reward" called ellagic acid, which creates a filter that reduces the "mutagenicity" of toxins entering our cells.[9] This matters because mutagens are chemical or physical agents capable of causing genetic alterations or mutations and damaging DNA, leading to cancer and other illnesses.

Beyond berries, knowledgeable foragers can collect mushrooms, wild carrots, fern fiddleheads, and herbs such as wild mint and sage. They can even gather seaweed! (Find out more on page 114 about using

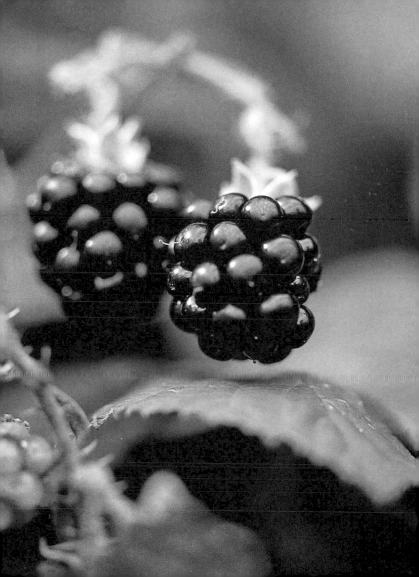

foraged seaweed.) My neighborhood still has remnants of the harvestable kitchen gardens that were there many years ago: An apple tree, a pear tree, a fig tree, plenty of mulberry trees, and some grapevines.

There are a couple of caveats before you start foraging, of course. First of all, be certain what you're putting into your mouth, especially when it comes to mushrooms, which can be highly poisonous. The best way to begin foraging is to go with someone who knows what they're doing. It may be a friend who has been living off their land for a long time, or someone who has dedicated themselves to studying the local flora. Look online for details of local foraging walks or groups. Second, consider the soil the plants are growing in, and make sure they haven't been exposed to toxic or bacteria-laden man- or animal-made substances.

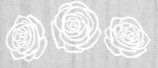

MARVELOUS MINT

The pleasure of an after-dinner mint began when the first forager plucked a leaf and enjoyed the menthol bite as well as the ease it brought to digestion. Mint is a primary herb that grows all over the world. There are over 25 species and 600 varieties of mint, including the perennial favorites peppermint and spearmint, although medicinally, peppermint tends to be more potent.

In the Middle East, particularly Morocco, mint tea—made with fresh mint, dried green tea, and lots of sugar—is prepared in a ceremonial manner, and is always offered to welcome guests. Refusing it is thought to be impolite. Tea bars are gathering places in the Middle East, much as cafes and pubs are in other parts of the world.

Mint is used to flavor many products, such as chewing gum and toothpaste, and the tea and volatile oil are reliable treatments for upset stomachs and related ailments. Mint calms the digestive muscles, as well as diminishing colds and headaches. In laboratory studies, it's been proven to kill some types of bacteria and viruses, suggesting that more research is merited.

Gathering Ginkgo

The ginkgo nut is a favorite of urban foragers. Why not try harvesting your own fruit in the fall? Wear rubber gloves in case you have a mild allergic reaction to them. You'll know the fruit is ripe if it smells a bit like vomit.

Soak the fruits overnight until you can separate out the nuts inside. After rinsing the nuts, spread them on a cookie sheet and bake at 180°F (80°C) for about 45 minutes—they're ready when the shells are dry. Store them in an airtight container for weeks or toast them right away in a cast-iron skillet with a little oil and salt. Crack the shells and eat the nuts inside—they taste a bit like chestnuts. Don't eat more than six or seven per day—too many can be toxic—and never give them to small children.

If you look the right way, you can see that the whole world is a garden.

Frances Hodgson Burnett, *The Secret Garden* (1911)

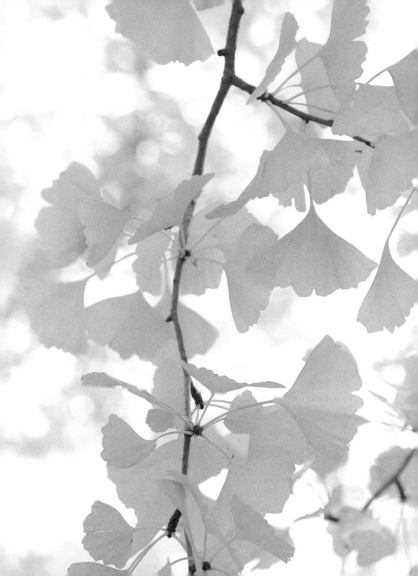

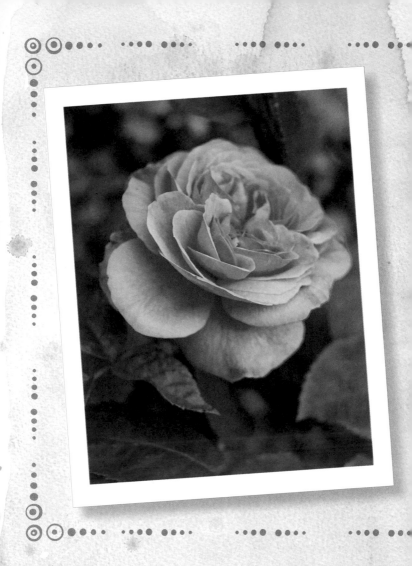

Chapter 5

Engaging Your Senses

The Sense of Nature

Recent studies by the noted social scientist Peter Aspinall of Heriot-Watt University, Edinburgh, and his colleagues have demonstrated that walking through urban green space elevated brain electroencephalogram (EEG) readings, lowering frustration and heightening engagement, and had an especially healing impact on older adults.[1] One can't help but wonder whether this effect is caused by the absence of city stress or something else. Maybe it has more to do with what the subjects are seeing—the green—than with where they are?

In 1984, Dr. Roger Ulrich (see page 129) published research in the journal *Science* that linked nature and healing.[2] He found that hospital patients who had plants in their rooms or even just looked at photographs of nature recovered much more quickly from surgery and required fewer painkillers. Perhaps this explains why we feel compelled to bring flowers to people who are sick. The blossoms brighten things up and immediately change the tone of the environment. They might be accompanied by a pleasing smell, but their uplifting effect seems to be primarily visual. As my neighbor Audra Tsanos, whose garden is a thing of wonder and delight in almost every season, puts it, "The eye seeks green." Nature produces a visual experience of infinite complexity and subtlety.

I go to nature to be soothed
and healed, and to have my
senses put in order.

John Burroughs (1837–1921)

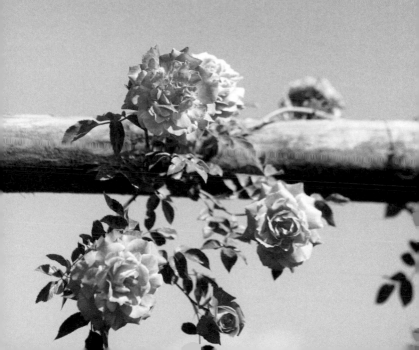

Seeing Colors

When we look at an object, it reflects light, which is received by the cells in our retinas, producing messages that are interpreted by the brain as images, colors, intensity, and so on. In the back of the eye, rods process light and dark and cones process the varying wavelengths that are perceived as color. Our brains are directly affected by what we see; there is a short but critical path between our eyes and our brain, and different parts of the brain hold different information: Faces, motion, distance, luminance.

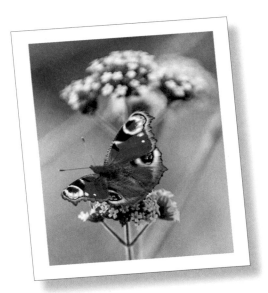

In her book *Healing Spaces*, Esther M. Sternberg asks: "Is there something about the structure of a scene that might be intrinsically jarring or relaxing—that could change your mood or affect healing?" She answers the question by explaining that there is a pathway from the visual cortex—the part of our brain that receives and processes sensory nerve impulses from the eyes—to the parahippocampal place area, which recognizes and recalls environmental scenes (such as landscapes) over other stimuli (such as faces). That's interesting, but this is amazing: "The nerve cells along this pathway express an increasing density of receptors of endorphins—the brain's own morphine-like molecules."[3]

Think of the possibilities: We might be able to heal ourselves simply by looking at images from nature! Sternberg goes on to explain how beautiful natural tableaux such as sunsets or misty forests have been shown to stimulate this opiating pathway. Remarkably, the more the nerve cells are stimulated by motion, color, and a variety of depths of perspective, the more active and opiating the release of endorphins becomes. Perhaps this evolved as a survival tool: The more that primitive people could see as they scanned the horizon, the more useful and potentially life-saving information they could gather. We have become what the neuroscientist Dr. Edward Vessel of the Max Planck Institute for Empirical Aesthetics calls "infovores," using visual information both to ascertain risk and to spark "cognitive pleasure."[4]

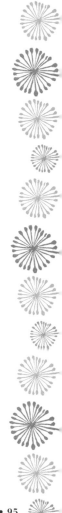

NOT ONLY GREEN

Green is not the only color to which we have an instinctive reaction. The longer the wavelength of the colors we're looking at (reds and oranges, rather than blues), the better we think. Studies at Rockefeller University, New York, have shown that our alertness and cognitive abilities are enhanced when we are exposed to orange light, as opposed to blue, which has a shorter wavelength.[5] This might be why we may grow dreamier when looking at a blue sky, but are drawn to and thrilled by sunsets.

PLANT POWER

A body of research undertaken by Japanese scientists in 2016 revealed that simply seeing fresh flowers (not even smelling or touching them) has calming effects. Chorong Song and her colleagues assembled a group of 114 people of varying ages, genders, and occupations, and had each person look at a bouquet of pink odorless roses for four minutes. By analyzing the participants' pulses, the scientists concluded that the visual stimulation of looking at the roses increased parasympathetic nervous activity, fostering a state of relaxation, while simultaneously decreasing sympathetic nervous activity and alleviating stress.[6]

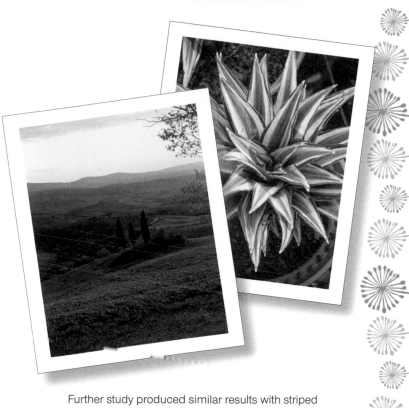

Further study produced similar results with striped *Dracaena* or corn plants. Even more studies have shown that we experience a calming response from observing three-dimensional plants and flowers—even if they are artificial—in lieu of photographs.[7] In other words, the real thing is best, artificial the second-best choice, but even photographs of fauna will produce some positive effects.

The Scents of Nature

The healing effects of being in nature do not just concern vision—they also involve smells. A great many studies have explored how smell influences our thinking. In particular, essential oils and other forms of fragrance can have a positive effect on how we remember and pay attention, on our self-confidence and experience of pain, and on how we make decisions.[8] This should sound pretty familiar to people who have tried aromatherapy, and there is a science to it. For example, it's been tested and shown that people who inhale the fragrance of rose oil feel calmer, more relaxed, and dreamier than those in a control group who don't. This has led to further research into the use of rose fragrance in treating or abating depression and anxiety.[9]

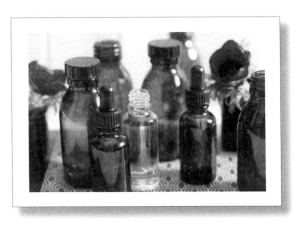

Of course, it's not just about roses. As we learned through forest bathing, the smell of pine woods and phytoncides—those volatile organic compounds that boost immune function—have a beneficial effect on our bodies and minds.

DISTINCTIVE CAMPHOR

As early as the Middle Ages, traders went in search of camphor in the tree's native Sumatra, Indonesia, China, and Borneo, and a distillation of the bark was used as an antiseptic and a treatment during influenza and cholera epidemics. In the 13th century, the Venetian Marco Polo referred to camphor in his journals, while in his *Complete History of Drugs* (1748), the French pharmacist Pierre Pomet wrote, "The Oil is very valuable for the Cure of Fevers, a Piece of Scarlet Cloth has been dipt [*sic*] into it being hung about the neck." There's a revered old camphor tree in Atami, Japan and it is said that each circumnavigation of the tree will add a year to your life.

It is with camphor's fragrance, though, that most of us connect. Crushing the leaves releases a pungent, spicy odor. Today, the essential oil is used in aromatherapy, as well as in ointments to relieve congestion and muscle pain, although in the past it was believed to ward off snakes and even evil spirits. The tree's wood and shoots can be put through a distillation process, transforming them into a crystalline white powder that looks like snow and is used in massage creams and astringents.

SWEET LINDEN

The fragrance of linden, or lime, blossoms, which cover the trees from June through August, is the stuff of sense memories and poetry. Brooklyn herbalist Cheryl Boiko put it like this when I asked her about linden flowers: "I love when I'm out and about in late spring ... and suddenly my senses are filled with the most delightful, light, sweet fragrance—it always takes me by surprise. I stop and look around and most often I find myself standing under a fully blooming linden tree with the little creamy-white clusters of flowers looking down at me." She went on to explain how the honey from the linden blossoms is a wonderful heart tonic, reducing blood pressure, cholesterol, and plaque, and can also lift the spirits in times of grief. It soothes coughs, can relieve cold and flu symptoms, and, because it is a mild sedative, it can help to ease tension headaches.

Sound Therapy

According to a study undertaken in 2018 by the Brighton and Sussex Medical School (BSMS) in the south of England, hearing sounds from nature, such as the roar of the ocean, helps us to focus our attention and allows us to relax.[10] You're not making it up when you feel as though the burble of running water, sparrows chirping, or the rustling of prairie grass relaxes you.

BSMS collaborated with the audiovisual artist Mark Ware to study what happened when people listened to recordings of natural and artificial sounds. Using an MRI scanner, they gauged brain activity while monitoring infinitesimal changes in heart rate. They learned that natural sounds increased brain connectivity and directed attention outward, whereas artificial sounds focused attention inward, creating a state similar to anxiety, depression, or PTSD.[11] This is unsurprising; I can't imagine that anyone wouldn't feel calmer listening to the rustling of trees or a stream than to traffic or construction sounds.

Even listening to natural sounds played on headphones increases parasympathetic activation, promoting and sustaining a sense of rest and counteracting stress. In a study published in the *International Journal of Environmental Research and Public Health* in 2010, university students exposed to natural sounds such as fountains and birdsong, rather than traffic noise, dealt better with a stressor (an arithmetic test).[12] There are long-term health benefits of diminished stress, so maybe it's time to dig out all those nature CDs or download a few tracks of whale calls or soothing rain rhythms—or maybe even record your own. Turn off your screens and try listening to sounds like this before going to sleep. (If you're in the city, try playing a recording at low volume.)

Sound has such a potent effect on us that some people think we should be aware of it in the same way as we monitor what we eat, drink, or breathe. After all, it's effectively another substance that we're putting into our bodies.

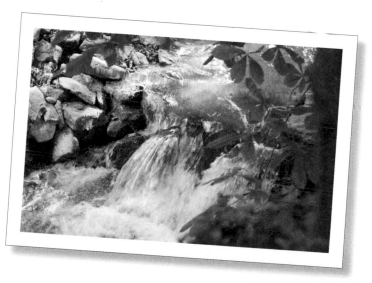

BIRDSONG

Birdsong has been found to be particularly restorative. Julian Treasure, author of *Sound Business* (2006), has said that birdsong evokes a state that he calls "body relaxed, mind alert." In 2013, he told the BBC: "People find birdsong relaxing and reassuring because over thousands of years they have learnt [that] when the birds sing they are safe, [and] it's when birds stop singing that people need to worry. Birdsong is also nature's alarm clock, with the dawn chorus signalling the start of the day, so it stimulates us cognitively." Treasure has put this to good use in a free smartphone app called Study, which claims to be a "productivity-boosting" soundscape to listen to while you work. He says it can help you to focus, improve cognition, and reduce tiredness. It's also intended to mask background noise—particularly conversation—that can disturb your concentration.[13]

Birdsong brings relief to my longing.
I am just as ecstatic as they are,
but with nothing to say.

Rumi (1207–1273)

SILENCE

Just as sounds can be healing, so is silence. Although it is hard to come by, most of us would agree that quiet is essential. Think about noise pollution, blaring screens, even the sometimes desirable background of white noise. All of it can lead to stress, sleeplessness, and more. We seek out earplugs and noise-canceling headphones for temporary respite, because it's easier to relax, think, and create without the stress and disruption of noise. Our world seems to be getting louder—with more traffic, cellphone pings and buzzes, televisions in waiting rooms, and music piped in everywhere—so seeking silence can be a challenge.

Traditional Japanese gardens include specific sense components, so that they address all means of perception, including sound. Running water is often incorporated, not just because it is perceived as cleansing, but also because its gentle sound contrasts with and enhances the silence.[14] How many times have you been able to solve a problem or clarify a situation after you've had a quiet moment to sort it out? That's where silence comes in, when the television is off, when you're all alone, or the moment at a crowded party or on a busy railroad station when suddenly everything falls still.

Sense Meditation

A famous exercise popularized by Jon Kabat-Zinn and taught in Mindfulness Stress Reduction Programs uses the contemplation and deliberate consumption of a single raisin to increase presence in mindfulness meditation.[15] Here I've adapted it to a dandelion flower, but you can use anything from nature—a pine cone, a blade of grass. See if you enjoy the healing effects of deeply experiencing a small bit of nature.

1 When out for a walk in nature, find a comfortable, quiet place to sit. Wherever it is, make sure it's a spot that allows you to get as quiet and as connected as possible to some aspect of nature.

····◉◎◉····

2 Pause and assess how you feel. Are you anxious? Tired? Restless? Bleary? Make a mental note of the sensation.

····◉◎◉····

3 Now, pick up the dandelion or whatever you're using for your meditation and weigh it in the palm of your hand. Feel its heft or lightness. Is it soft? Sticky?

4 Next, look at it. Really focus on it with your complete attention. Imagine it's the first dandelion you've ever seen. Can you find any fractal patterns (see page 40)? What does the color yellow evoke for you?

••••⊙◎◎••••

5 Turn the flower over between your fingers and connect to its texture and feel. Try closing your eyes, so that all your information comes solely from touch.

••••⊙◎◎••••

6 Try smelling the dandelion. Is there a fragrance? Is it pleasant or unpleasant? Assuming you're not allergic, don't just sniff it, but hold it near your nose and breathe slowly and deeply. Repeat for a few breaths.

••••⊙◎◎••••

7 Now, close your eyes and picture the dandelion. What does it evoke for you? Look at that thought and let it go as you assess how you feel. Are you more relaxed? Do you feel focused? Is there a sense of being more connected to your surroundings?

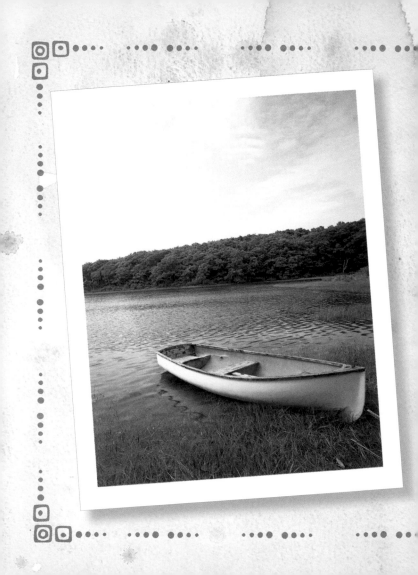

Chapter 6
Water Treatment

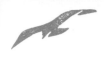

Seeing the Sea

Numerous scientific studies support the idea that just being near a body of water, like being near a green space, is good for body and mind. For example, analysis in 2012 by the University of Exeter, in southwest England, found that the closer people lived to the coast, the healthier they tended to be. The researchers also learned that—as with green spaces—the positive impact was especially notable among less affluent socio-economic groups who have fewer opportunities to live near the sea or take vacations there, leading them to find a correlation between life near the shore, lowered stress, and increased exercise.[1]

It's unsurprising, as we're endlessly fascinated by and connected to water. For example, some 270 million visits are made to English coastlines each year, which is remarkable for a country with a population of 66 million.[2] As Wallace J. Nichols, founder of Ocean Revolution, wrote in his brilliant book *Blue Mind: How Water Makes You Happier, More Connected, and Better at What You Do* (2014), "Water is changing all the time, but it's also fundamentally familiar. It seems to entertain our brains nicely with novelty plus a soothing regular background."[3]

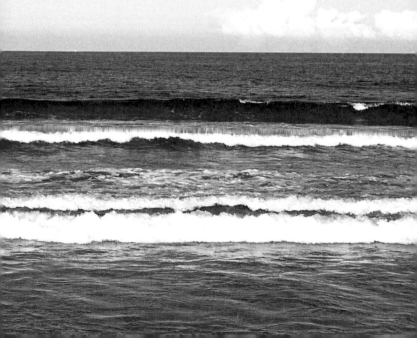

Water purifies and regenerates because it nullifies the past, and restores—even if only for a moment—the integrity of the dawn of things.

Mircea Eliade, *Patterns in Comparative Religion* (1958)[4]

BLUE VIEWS

We have already learned about the effect of views of greenery (see page 92), but some studies have considered how seeing water scenes or "blue" environments can affect our health. Researchers at the universities of Exeter and Plymouth, in southwest England, studied the physical and psychological effects of urban (gray), park and woodland (green), and river and coastline (blue) views on post-menopausal women as they rode stationary bikes for 15 minutes.[5] The affective results—mood and feelings—for the green scenes were similar to those found in the other studies, and generally low for the urban environments (no surprise there), but the cyclists who were looking at blue scenes reported that the time seemed to go faster and they were more willing to keep exercising.[6]

Fortunately for the 60% of us who don't live near a coastline, even periodic visits can help us to flourish.[7] Researchers from Kobe University in Japan affirm that visits to natural environments can reduce stress and provide a sense of restoration, healing the body as we heal the mind. They also found that merely living near the beach isn't as helpful as stopping to take the time to appreciate the ocean view. Interestingly, there is a bigger impact on women than on men. Their experience of gazing at the sea induced feelings of grandeur, awe, peace of mind, and enchantment.

Scientists have linked this understanding to aquariums as well as to ocean views.[8] Research was conducted at the National Marine Aquarium in Plymouth, southwest England, to find out if looking at biota (plant and animal life) in water affected physical and psychological wellbeing. The heart rate and mood of visitors to the aquarium were monitored as they looked at tanks containing only seawater, at partially stocked tanks, and at fully stocked tanks of fish and marine vegetation. One of the researchers, Dr. Mathew P. White, pointed out: "The first thing to notice is that people relaxed, even watching an empty tank, and the benefits increased as we introduced more fish."[9] This response was especially positive when it came to lowering stress.

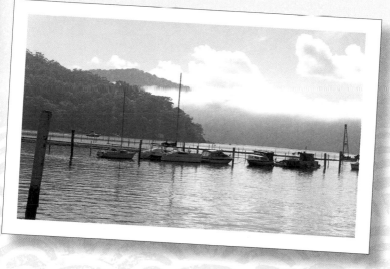

FORAGING SEAWEED

When walking by the coast, why not forage for seaweed? You can use seaweed for all sorts of things: It's a nutritious mulch for plants, great for thickening soups and seasoning stocks and salads, and can be a natural source of MSG, that savory umami taste.

Seaweed is a kind of algae, not a plant. It is high in protein, and contains vitamin B12, iodine, potassium, phosphorus, magnesium, sodium, and calcium.[10] Each of these is beneficial. Among other things, B12 encourages cell growth, iodine influences nerve and muscle function, potassium and sodium balance fluids in the body, phosphorus and calcium build bones and teeth, and magnesium regulates blood pressure.

Ocean seaweed is generally safe to consume—whereas most freshwater algae are toxic—but there are a few exceptions, such as lyngbya, featherweed, and acid kelp. There are more than 35,000 types of seaweed, so do some research and be absolutely certain what you're putting in your mouth or on your skin. (If you're in doubt, opt for store-bought!)

Three abundant, accessible, and easy options found in the Atlantic Ocean are laver, giant kelp, and sea lettuce.[11] I tried harvesting laver—which is similar to nori that is used in sushi and Japanese snacks—because it seemed the least intimidating, and its dark green color made it easy to spot. It's best to harvest seaweed in cooler weather, because by summer it's at the end of its growing season and the heat can cause it to rot.

- Make sure you're foraging from unpolluted water.

- Harvest living plants, not the seaweed that has washed ashore and is on the beach.

- Cut about 3–5 in. (7.5–12.5 cm) from the base.

- Wash thoroughly and as soon as possible (to free up any little sea creatures).

- Hang on a clothesline or drying rack in the sun for a few hours. It solidifies quickly!

- When it's dry, store it in a humidity-proof container.

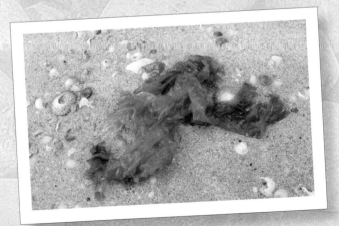

Take the Plunge

If you're near a body of water, try walking in it: It's better exercise than walking on land, because you are working against the water's resistance. This form of exercise is especially recommended for people with arthritis or limited abilities, for whom swimming laps is not a possibility. Plus, your feet get a nice massage as a bonus!

To fully experience the water's healing benefits, try taking a dip or a glide, if that's an option. It's common knowledge that swimming is great exercise, and so are boating and paddle-boarding. When we're on a board or in a kayak, not only are we moving our muscles and strengthening our lungs, we're also applying mental focus to stay upright—improving balance and concentration— and we're directly connected to the psychological healing of being with water.

I know the joy of fishes in the river through my own joy, as I go walking along the same river.

Chuang Tzu (late 4th century BCE)

FOOTBATHS

Most of us have experienced the relief that comes from soaking our feet after a long day of walking, standing, or exercising. We all know that standing at the edge of the sea and feeling the cool waves lap at our feet is soothing, and so is the cooling sensation of walking through a cold mountain stream or a clear lake.

Footbaths can soothe muscles and joints, but it turns out they may also ease our minds. Three times a week for four weeks, Japanese researchers gave footbaths and leg massages to psychiatric patients with schizophrenia, and measured the effects. The patients became more physically relaxed, but what's fascinating is that the treatment was also successful in ameliorating their psychiatric symptoms.[12]

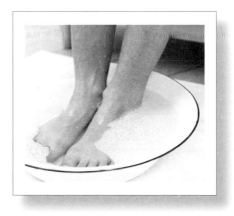

Chasing Waterfalls

Negative ions are oxygen ions with an extra electron attached, and can result from changes in weather conditions, so when it rains they're produced through water molecules. A downpour provides us with the benefit of negative ions and increases the flow of oxygen to the brain, producing biochemical reactions that raise serotonin, improving our mood and making us more alert. Other studies report that negative ions can facilitate the treatment of PTSD, addiction, and depression.[13]

According to researchers from Paracelsus Medical University in Salzburg, Austria, a wonderful way to get a generous dose of those positive vibes is by visiting a waterfall, especially one at high altitude.[14] The falling water amps up the ionization, creating an aerosol effect that has positive psychological effects, lowering stress, and boosts the immune system.

Even the wonderful sound of rushing water is relaxing. Some people suggest that it's because it replicates the sound we hear in the womb, but it may be because our brains interpret sounds as threats (think thunder or alarms) or comforts (think waves lapping at the shore), according to Orfeu Buxton, an associate professor of biobehavioral health at Pennsylvania State University. Repeated soothing sounds create a sense of ease. he says: "It's like they're saying: 'Don't worry, don't worry, don't worry.'"[15]

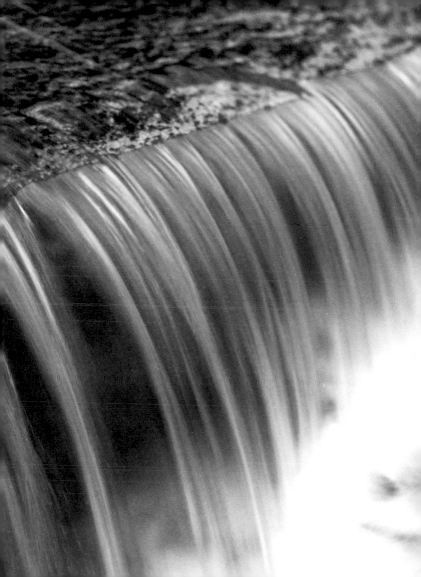

Water Meditation

Try a water-bowl offering based on a traditional Tibetan technique, taught by a Buddhist teacher trained in a Tibetan lineage and whom I work with and admire, Dr. Miles Neale.[16]

1 Gather seven small bowls or containers.

•••◉ ◎ ◉•••

2 Arrange them on an altar or in a place that has meaning for you, in a line, separated one from the other by the length of a grain of rice.

•••◉ ◎ ◉•••

3 Hold one of the bowls, fill it with water, and present it as an offering.

4 Pour water from the first bowl into the second, from the second into the third, and so on. As you do, imagine you're transforming the liquid step-by-step into these sacred materials:

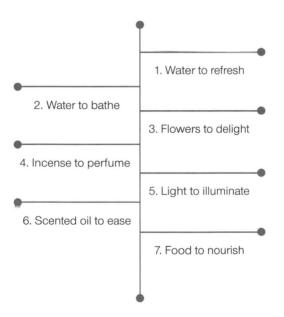

1. Water to refresh

2. Water to bathe

3. Flowers to delight

4. Incense to perfume

5. Light to illuminate

6. Scented oil to ease

7. Food to nourish

If you wish, you can incorporate sounds into your meditation—music, affirmations, prayers, or a mantra—or burn a candle to symbolize bringing light into the world.

Neale explains that the idea behind this practice "is based on the science of karmic causality—cause and effect—not dogma or rote. The power of creative imagination to influence our neurobiology is well documented, and so an ordinary act of offering water can be transformed into an extraordinary act of offering sacred substances. The brain registers the potency whether the action is real or imagined. The ritual then becomes a sacred skill training of openheartedness that optimally changes your mind and affects future perception."

In one drop of water are found
all the secrets of the oceans.

Kahlil Gibran (1883–1931)

Chapter 7
Open a Window

When We Cannot Take a Walk

No matter how much we wish to walk and connect with nature out in the world—in neighborhood parks or camping trips, botanic gardens, or even favorite cemeteries—there are times when it is simply not possible: For example, in times of illness, periods of inclement weather, and when juggling busy schedules. Fortunately, the act of simply opening a window can bring many of its own benefits.

Open a window right now. If you are in an office building or a rainstorm (or both) and can't open a window, at least sit by one. Take a deep breath. Look up into the sky or let your gaze settle on something green—a tree, a hedge, a flower bed, a potted plant. Take another breath.

Did you notice a shift? Chances are you slowed your heart rate, drew in a little more (probably cleaner) oxygen, which improved your focus and concentration, and gave your back a bit of a stretch. You gathered your thoughts and, even for the briefest of moments, felt part of the world beyond yourself—mindful and connected. Your mood may have improved. All this in less than a minute, and without a gadget, supplement, or special clothing or shoes! If that's not wonderful, I don't know what is.

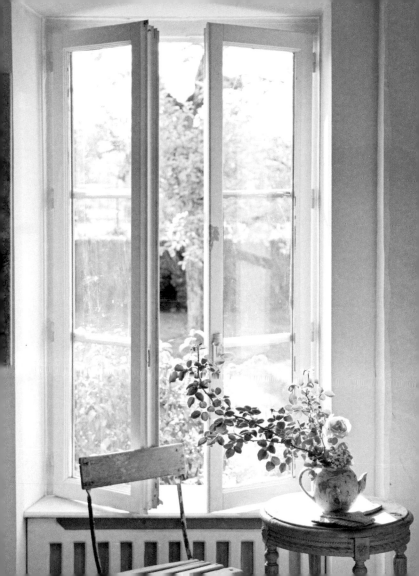

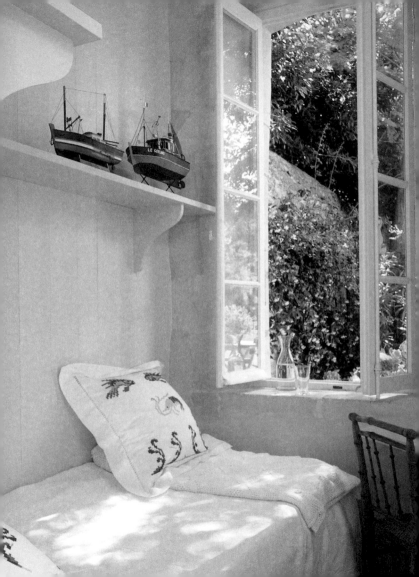

A ROOM WITH A VIEW

Dr. Roger S. Ulrich, Ph.D. EDAC, was a trailblazer in evidence-based healthcare design—the scientific relationship between a built environment and the impact it has on the people who use it. He was the first to gather and publish data on how merely looking through a window can help to heal us. He examined patients recovering from gallbladder removal surgery in a hospital in Pennsylvania between 1972 and 1981. Of the 200 patients he studied, 23 were assigned to rooms looking out on deciduous trees, while the others had a view of a brick wall. He published his results in an article, "View through a Window May Influence Recovery from Surgery":

"Twenty-three surgical patients assigned to rooms with windows looking out on a natural scene had shorter postoperative hospital stays, received fewer negative evaluative comments in nurses' notes, and took fewer potent analgesics than 23 matched patients in similar rooms with windows facing a brick building wall."[1]

Remarkable! As far as I can tell, Ulrich's study was the first formal one on this subject, but it has been supported by many since. One done with pulmonary patients in 2011 showed that by measuring mental health, subjective wellbeing, and emotional states, as well as other markers, "an unobstructed bedroom view to natural surroundings appears to have better supported improvement in self-reported physical and mental health."[2]

Natural Light

The restorative power of nature can be found not just in what we see through the window, but also in what comes in. Even if the weather is cold, pulling back the curtains or opening the blinds and giving yourself a break from artificial light can improve your state of mind. There is a genuine connection between how much daylight we are exposed to and how well we sleep. The neuroscientist Ivy Cheung, while doing post-doctoral work at Harvard Medical School's Division of Sleep Medicine, found that the amount of daylight that workers are exposed to has a remarkable impact, and for the sake of the wellness of employees we should consider how our office buildings (or any workplace) incorporate natural light.[3] This is because artificial light doesn't balance our circadian rhythms—our sleeping/waking cycles over a period of 24 hours—the way natural light does, and of course it doesn't apply solely to the workplace.

Looking out of a window and receiving light through it are both valuable, easy actions to take to improve our physical, psychological, and maybe even spiritual wellbeing, but the benefits multiply when we open those windows. Take vitamin D, for example. The human need for it has been well established, and a deficiency can lead to all sorts of medical problems such as malabsorption of nutrients and rickets, a softening of the bones. One of the

There is something
infinitely healing
in the repeated
refrains of nature—
the assurance that
dawn comes after
night, and spring
after the winter.

Rachel Carson, *The Sense
of Wonder* (1965)

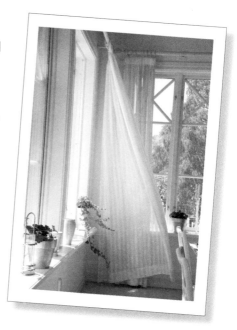

best ways to get vitamin D is through exposure to
sunlight, since the sun emits ultraviolet waves that set off
a chemical reaction when they reach the skin, creating
vitamin D. But the important thing is that although
sunshine can pass through glass, the ultraviolet waves
cannot, so if you want to increase your intake of vitamin
D, sit by an open window.

Fresh Air

There is more to an open window than vitamin absorption. When you were a child and your parents told you to go outside and get some fresh air, they were onto something. That's why the World Health Organization recommends fresh-air ventilation as a way to diminish the transmission of communicable diseases, such as COVID-19 and tuberculosis. Interviewed in *Scientific American*, the infection control specialist Rod Escombe of Imperial College London described a study he had carried out in Lima, Peru, in which he compared the airflow of 70 rooms in eight hospitals that treated tuberculosis patients. If windows and doors allowed air to flow, the air in a room was fully replaced about 28 times per hour—even more than if ventilation fans were used without open windows (only about 12 times per hour). Escombe recommended that waiting rooms have access to the outdoors, that hospitals have larger windows as well as skylights that can open, and that tuberculosis wards be downwind of other areas.[4]

Think about this in terms of your everyday life—perhaps not tuberculosis, but the common cold. You've probably noticed that you tend to get sick more often after spending time in an enclosed space with lots of people, such as in the cabin of an airplane, a classroom, or the doctor's waiting room. When air can't circulate, the odds of germs cycling and recycling through our systems increase exponentially. Bill Sothern, an expert in indoor air quality and the founder of Microecologies, told *The New York Times*: "The air indoors is 10 times more contaminated than the air outdoors at any given time."[5] This can lead to headaches, asthma, allergies, lethargy, and dermatological conditions in homes, schools, workplaces, hospitals, and anywhere else that people congregate.

So open that window, and do your best not to close it when you go to bed. We rest more deeply and for longer not just if we're exposed to natural light during the day, but also if there is a constant flow of fresh air during the night. A study published in the journal *Indoor Air* found that in ventilated spaces where the air circulates there is less carbon dioxide buildup. Although it is crucial for many things (including photosynthesis of plants), carbon dioxide is the gas that we exhale, flushing impurities from our bodies. Lower carbon dioxide levels in the air around us lead to deeper, longer, and less interrupted sleep.[6] Our bodies don't have to work so hard to do their jobs of cleansing our cells, lungs, and blood, and so we can better settle and rest.

Fostering Connection

When we look out of a window, we get out of our own heads and connect with the world beyond the self. Sometimes we have no time to engage with other people, but it can be healing to know that they are there. Looking out of a window in the city and seeing your fellow humans can create a sense of connection, commonality, and compassion: Perhaps they are going through a difficult time ... they found love ... they survived childhood ... they're tired after a long day at work—just like us.

Observing nature can foster a similar feeling of interconnection. It can make our problems feel smaller and give us context within the vastness of the universe, a sense of peace and awe. When I think of the times I have felt most spiritually connected, they have not been dramatic or calculated—at retreats or organized events— but in small moments of perception: The whisper of a breeze through the trees, a startlingly blue sky, the sudden appearance of ducklings out of tall grass.

Try making window time into a daily meditation for yourself. It is one of the simplest and yet most reliable self-care practices you are likely ever to find—this tiny action can change your mood, your day, your way of being. Think of window time as a formal practice, not just a random event.

1 Purposefully and mindfully take 30 seconds to gaze out of the window. It can be a kitchen window or a train window, looking onto a forest, a single sapling, or up to the sky, no matter—with active intention and attention, do that one thing: Look out of the window.

2 Try it for a few days. You may find it helpful to create a reminder for yourself. I set the alarm on my phone, but you might prefer to connect the action mentally to specific points in the day, such as after you have eaten a meal or as soon as you arrive at work or school.

3 Pay attention to any changes during your window time meditation, and later in the day. Do you notice a positive result?

Notes

Chapter 1: Take a Walk

1 Howard V. Hong and Edna H. Hong, *The Essential Kierkegaard* (Princeton University Press, 2013), p. 502.

2 "Sitting Is Bad for Your Brain: Not Just Your Metabolism or Heart," *Science Daily*, April 12, 2018, www.sciencedaily.com/releases/2018/04/180412141014.htm.

3 C.E. Matthews et al., "Amount of Time Spent in Sedentary Behaviors and Cause-specific Mortality in US Adults," *American Journal of Clinical Nutrition*, 95/2 (2012), pp. 437–45, www.ncbi.nlm.nih.gov/pubmed/22218159.

4 Jill K. Morris et al., "Aerobic Exercise for Alzheimer's Disease: A Randomized Controlled Pilot Trial," *PLoS One*, 12/2 (February 10, 2017), www.journals.plos.org/plosone/article?id=10.1371/journal.pone.0170547.

5 Esther M. Sternberg, *Healing Spaces* (Belknap Press, 2009).

6 Byambaa Enkhmaa et al., "Lifestyle Changes: Effect of Diet, Exercise, Functional Food, and Obesity Treatment on Lipids and Lipoproteins," *Endotext*, June 8, 2015, www.ncbi.nlm.nih.gov/books/NBK326737.

7 Melissa R. Marselle et al., "Moving beyond Green: Exploring the Relationship of Environment Type and Indicators of Perceived Environmental Quality on Emotional Well-Being following Group Walks," *International Journal of Environmental Research and Public Health*, 12/1 (2015), pp. 106–130.

8 Gregory N. Bratman et al., "Nature Experience Reduces Rumination and Subgenual Prefrontal Cortex Activation," *Proceedings of the National Academy of Sciences of the United States of America*, 112/28 (July 14, 2015), www.pnas.org/content/112/28/8567.

9 Johannes Michalak et al., "How We Walk Affects What We Remember: Gait Modifications Through Biofeedback Change Negative Memory Bias," *Journal of Behavior Therapy and Experimental Psychiatry*, 46 (March 2015), pp. 121–25, quoted in "How To Feel Better By Just Walking Differently," *PsyBlog*, October 19, 2014, www.spring.org.uk/2014/10/how-to-feel-happy-just-bywalking-differently.php.

10 "Going Outside—Even in the Cold—Improves Memory, Attention," *Michigan News*, University of Michigan, December 16, 2008, www.news.umich.edu/going-outsideeven-in-thecoldimproves-memory-attention.

11 Gregory N. Bratman et al., "Nature Experience Reduces Rumination and Subgenual Prefrontal Cortex Activation," *Proceedings of the National Academy of Sciences of the United States of America*, 112/28 (July 14, 2015), www.pnas.org/content/112/28/8567.

12 May Wong, "Stanford Study Finds Walking Improves Creativity," *Stanford News*, April 24, 2014, https://news.stanford.edu/2014/04/24/walking-vs-sitting-042414.

13 Clark Strand, *Waking Up to the Dark* (Spiegel & Grau, 2015), p. 17.

14 Thich Nhat Hanh, *Present Moment, Wonderful Moment* (Parallax Press, 2002), p. 57.

Chapter 2: Forest Bathing

1 Ahmad Hassan et al., "Effects of Walking in Bamboo Forest and City Environments on Brainwave Activity in Young Adults," *Evidence-based Complementary and Alternative Medicine*, 2018, www.hindawi.com/journals/ecam/2018/9653857.

2 "Immerse Yourself in a Forest for Better Health," New York State Department of Environmental Conservation, www.dec.ny.gov/lands/90720.html, accessed August 2018.; Gen Xiang Mao et al., "Additive Benefits of Twice Forest Bathing Trips in Elderly Patients with Chronic Heart Failure," *Biomedical and Environmental Sciences*, 31/2 (February 2018), www.ncbi.nlm.nih.gov/pubmed/29606196.

3 Kyoung Sang Cho et al., "Terpenes from Forests and Human Health," *Toxicology Research*, 33/2 (April 2017), pp. 97–106, www.ncbi.nlm.nih.gov/pubmed/28443180.

4 Qing Li, *Forest Bathing* (Penguin, 2018).

5 Richard Taylor, "Fractal Patterns in Nature and Art Are Aesthetically Pleasing and Stress-reducing," *The Conversation*, March 31, 2017, www.theconversation.com/fractal-patterns-innature-and-art-are-aesthetically-pleasing-and-stress-reducing-73255.

6 Quoted in Diane Toomey, "How Listening to Trees Can Help Reveal Nature's Connections," *Yale Environment 360*, August 24, 2017, www.e360.yale.edu/features/how-listening-to-trees-can-help-reveal-natures-connections.

7 Richard Grant, "Do Trees Talk to Each Other?," *Smithsonian*, March 2018, www.smithsonianmag.com/science-nature/thewhispering-trees-180968084.

8 See www.greencitysolutions.de/en/solutions.

Chapter 3: Delightful Dirt

1 James L. Oschman et al., "The Effects of Grounding (Earthing) on Inflammation, the Immune Response, Wound Healing, and Prevention and Treatment of Chronic Inflammatory and Autoimmune Diseases," *Journal of Inflammation Research*, 8 (March 24, 2015), pp. 83–96, www.ncbi.nlm.nih.gov/pmc/articles/PMC4378297.

2 Antygona Chadzopulu et al., "The Therapeutic Effects of Mud," *Progressive Health Sciences*, 1/2 (2011), www.nymedicalcare.com/Docs/mud.pdf.

3 Hagit Matz, Edith Orion, and Ronni Wolf, "Balneotherapy in Dermatology," *Dermatologic Therapy*, 16 (2003), pp. 132–40, www.sld.cu/galerias/pdf/sitios/rehabilitacion-bal/matzh_et_al.pdf.

4 M.E. O'Brien et al., "SRL172 (Killed Mycobacterium vaccae) in Addition to Standard Chemotherapy Improves Quality of Life Without Affecting Survival, in Patients with Advanced Non-small-cell Lung Cancer: Phase III Results," *Annals of Oncology*, 15/6 (June 2004), pp. 906–14, www.ncbi.nlm.nih.gov/pubmed/15151947.

5 Jenni Laidman, "Microbes Rule Your Health—and Further Prove that Kids Should Eat Dirt," *Chicago Tribune*, October 13, 2017, www.chicagotribune.com/lifestyles/health/sc-hlth-microbiome-1018-story.html.

6 Linda Chen, "The Old and Mysterious Practice of Eating Dirt, Revealed," *NPR*, April 2, 2014, www.npr.org/sections/thesalt/2014/04/02/297881388/the-old-and-mysteriouspractice-of-eating-dirt-revealed.

7 Lisa Elaine Held, "5 Foods That Have More Potassium Than a Banana," *Well+Good*, September 15, 2011, www.wellandgood.com/good-advice/5-foods-that-have-morepotassium-than-a-banana.

8 Ruairi Robertson, "10 Ways to Improve Your Gut Bacteria, Based on Science," *Healthline*, November 18, 2016, www.healthline.com/nutrition/improve-gut-bacteria#section5.

9 *Ibid*.

10 Elise Alvaro et al., "Composition and Metabolism of the Intestinal Microbiota in Consumers and Non-consumers of Yogurt," *British Journal of Nutrition*, 97/1 (January 2007), www.ncbi.nlm.nih.gov/pubmed/17217568.

Chapter 4: Being in Nature

1 Tyra A. Olstad, *Zen of the Plains: Experiencing Wild Western Places* (University of North Texas Press, 2014), p. 235.

2 Jill Neimark, "Extreme Chemical Sensitivity Makes Sufferers Allergic to Life," *Discover*, December 11, 2013, www.discovermagazine.com/2013/nov/13-allergic-life.

3 Petter Erik Leirhaug, "The Role of *Friluftsliv* in Henrik Ibsen's Works," paper delivered at "Henrik Ibsen: The Birth of '*Friluftsliv*': A 150-Year International Dialogue Conference Jubilee Celebration," North Troendelag University College, Norway, September 14–19, 2009, www.norwegianjournaloffriluftsliv.com/doc/172010.pdf.

4 Luke (Natural Resources Institute Finland), "The Effects of Nature on Well-Being," www.luke.fi/en/natural-resources/recreational-use-of-nature/the-effects-of-nature-well-being, accessed August 2018.

5 Magdalena M.H.E. van den Berg et al., "Autonomic Nervous System Responses to Viewing Green and Built Settings: Differentiating Between Sympathetic and Parasympathetic Activity," *International Journal of Environmental Research and Public Health*, 12/12 (December 2015), pp. 15,860–74, www.ncbi.nlm.nih.gov/pmc/articles/PMC4690962.

6 CIRIA, "Psychological," www.opengreenspace.com/opportunities-and-challenges/health/psychological, accessed August 2018.

7 "Why Green Spaces Are Good for Gray Matter," *Neuroscience News*, April 10, 2017, www.neurosciencenews.com/green-spaces-neurobiology-6376.

8 Robin Wall Kimmerer, *Braiding Sweetgrass* (Milkweed Editions, 2014), p. 10.

9 Diana Beresford-Kroeger, *The Sweetness of a Simple Life* (Vintage Canada, 2015) p. 77.

Chapter 5: Engaging Your Senses

1 Peter Aspinall et al., "The Urban Brain: Analysing Outdoor Physical Activity with Mobile EEG," *British Journal of Sports Medicine*, 49/4 (February 2015), pp. 272–76, www.ncbi.nlm.nih.gov/pubmed/23467965; Chris Neale et al., "The Ageing Urban Brain: Analyzing Outdoor Physical Activity Using the Emotiv Affectiv Suite in Older People," *Journal of Urban Health*, 94/6 (December 2017), pp. 869–80, https://link.springer.com/article/10.1007/s11524-017-0191-9.

2 R. S. Ulrich, "View Through a Window May Influence Recovery from Surgery," *Science*, 224/4647 (April 27, 1984), pp. 420–421.

3 Esther M. Sternberg, *Healing Spaces* (Belknap Press, 2009).

4 Edward A. Vessel and Irving Biedermann, "Why Do We Prefer Looking at Some Scenes Rather than Others?," talk presented at OPAM, a conference on Object Perception and Memory, 2001, www.cns.nyu.edu/~vessel/pubs/Vessel_OPAM2001_print.pdf.

5 Sarah Laxhmi Chellappa et al., "Photic Memory for Executive Brain Responses," *Proceedings of the National Academy of Sciences*, 111/16 (April 22, 2014): pp. 6087-091, www.pnas.org/content/111/16/6087.

6 Chorong Song, Harumi Ikei, and Yoshifumi Miyazaki, "Physiological Effects of Nature Therapy: A Review of the Research in Japan," *International Journal of Environmental Research and Public Health*, 13/8 (August 2016), p. 781, www.ncbi.nlm.nih.gov/pmc/articles/PMC4997467.

7 Sarah Laxhmi Chellappa et al., "Photic Memory for Executive Brain Responses," *Proceedings of the National Academy of Sciences*, 111/16 (April 22, 2014): pp. 6087-091, www.pnas.org/content/111/16/6087.

8 Andrew J. Johnson, "Cognitive Facilitation Following Intentional Odor Exposure," *Sensors*, 11/5 (2011), pp. 5469–88, www.ncbi.nlm.nih.gov/pubmed/22163909.

9 Tapanee Hongratanaworakit, "Relaxing Effect of Rose Oil on Humans," *Natural Product Communications*, 4/2 (February 2009), pp. 291–96, www.ncbi.nlm.nih.gov/pubmed/19370942.

10 Cassandra D. Gould van Praag et al., "Mind-wandering and Alterations to Default Mode Network Connectivity When Listening to Naturalistic Versus Artificial Sounds," *Scientific Reports*, 7 (2017), www.nature.com/articles/srep45273.

11 "How the Sounds of Nature Help Us to Relax," *Neuroscience News*, March 30, 2017, www.neurosciencenews.com/nature-sound-relaxation-6311.

12 Jesper J. Alvarsson, Stefan Wiens, and Mats E. Nilsson, "Stress Recovery During Exposure to Nature Sound and Environmental Noise," *International Journal of Environmental Research and Public Health*, 7/3 (March 2010), pp. 1036–46, www.ncbi.nlm.nih.gov/pmc/articles/PMC2872309.

13 Denise Winterman, "The Surprising Uses for Birdsong," *BBC News*, May 8, 2013, www.bbc.com/news/magazine-22298779.

14 George Prochnik, *In Pursuit of Silence* (Doubleday Books, 2010), p. 237.

15 "Raisin Meditation," https://ggia.berkeley.edu/practice/raisin_meditation#

Chapter 6: Water Treatment

1 Benedict W. Wheeler et al., "Does Living by the Coast Improve Health and Wellbeing?," *Health & Place*, 18/5 (September 2012), pp. 1198–1201, www.doi.org/10.1016/j.healthplace.2012.06.015.

2 "270 Million Visits Made to English Coastlines Each Year," *Science Daily*, April 5, 2018, www.sciencedaily.com/releases/2018/04/180405120359.htm.

3 Wallace J. Nichols, *Blue Mind* (Little, Brown 2014), p. 155.

4 Mircea Eliade, *Patterns in Comparative Religion* (1958), p. 194.

5 Mathew P. White et al., "The Effects of Exercising in Different Natural Environments on Psycho-Physiological Outcomes in Post-Menopausal Women: A Simulation Study," *International Journal of Environmental Research and Public Health*, 12 (2015), pp. 11,929–53, https://pdfs.semanticscholar.org /45f2/9b7fdf1552d2ca523c35b96dffdc17c.pdf.

6 *Ibid.*

7 "Percentage of Total Population Living in Coastal Areas," United Nations, www.un.org/esa/sustdev/natlinfo/indicators/methodology_sheets/oceans_seas_coasts/pop_coastal_areas.pdf.

8 Deborah Cracknell et al., "Marine Biota and Psychological Well-Being: A Preliminary Examination of Dose-Response Effects in an Aquarium Setting," *Environment and Behavior*, 48/10 (December 2016), pp. 1242–69, http://journals.sagepub.com/doi/abs/10.1177/0013916515597512.

9 Quoted in Mark Kinver, "Aquariums 'Deliver Significant Health Benefits,'" *BBC News*, July 30, 2015, www.bbc.com/news/science-environment-33716589.

10 Eun-Sun Hwang, Kyung-Nam Ki, and Ha-Yull Chang, "Proximate Composition, Amino Acid, Mineral, and Heavy Metal Content of Dried Laver," *Preventive Nutrition and Food Science*, 18/2 (June 2013), pp. 139–44, www.ncbi.nlm.nih.gov/pmc/articles/PMC3892503.

11 "Where to Harvest Seaweed and How to Eat It," *Forage SF*, October 14, 2015, www.foragesf.com/blog/2015/10/14/where-to-harvest-seaweed-and-how-to-eat-it.

12 Kazuko Kito and Keiko Suzuki, "Research on the Effect of the Foot Bath and Foot Massage on Residual Schizophrenia Patients," *Archives of Psychiatric Nursing*, 30/3 (June 2016), pp. 375–81, www.sciencedirect.com/science/article/pii/S0883941716000030.

13 Vanessa Perez, Dominik D. Alexander, and William H. Bailey, "Air Ions and Mood Outcomes: A Review and Meta-analysis," *BMC Psychiatry*, 13 (2013), p. 29, www.ncbi.nlm.nih.gov/pmc/articles/PMC3598548.

14 Carina Grafetstätter et al., "Does Waterfall Aerosol Influence Mucosal Immunity and Chronic Stress? A Randomized Controlled Clinical Trial," *Journal of Physiological Anthropology*, 36/10 (2017), www.ncbi.nlm.nih.gov/pmc/articles/PMC5237191.

15 Quoted in Adam Hadhazy, "Why Does the Sound of Water Help You Sleep?," *Live Science*, January 18, 2016, www.livescience.com/53403-why-sound-of-water-helps-you-sleep.html.

16 "Water Meditation" adapted from *Gradual Awakening: The Tibetan Buddhist Path of Becoming Fully Human*, by Miles Neale PsyD, copyright 2018, Boulder, Colorado: Sounds True. Reprinted and adapted with permission of the author.

Chapter 7: Open a Window

1 Roger S. Ulrich, "View Through a Window May Influence Recovery from Surgery," *Science*, 224/4647 (April 27, 1984), pp. 420–1.

2 Ruth Kjærsti Raanaas et al., "Health Benefits of a View of Nature Through the Window: A Quasi-Experimental Study of Patients in a Residential Rehabilitation Center," *Clinical Rehabilitation*, 26/1 (2012), pp. 21–32, www.ncbi.nlm.nih.gov/pubmed/21856720.

3 Christopher Bergland, "Exposure to Natural Light Improves Workplace Performance," *Psychology Today* blog, June 5, 2013, www.psychologytoday.com/us/blog/the-athletes-way/201306/exposure-natural-light-improves-workplace-performance.

4 J.R. Minkel, "A Breath of Fresh Air: To Fight Tuberculosis, Open a Window," *Scientific American*, February 26, 2007, www.scientificamerican.com/article/a-breath-of-fresh-air-to.

5 Quoted in Robin Finn, "Mold, Come Out with Your Hands Up," *New York Times*, May 3, 2013, www.nytimes.com/2013/05/05/realestate/bill-sothern-remediates-mold-and-other-hazards.html.

6 Carolyn Crist, "Open Windows and Doors Can Improve Sleep Quality," *Reuters*, December 7, 2017, www.reuters.com/article/ushealth-sleep/open-windows-and-doors-can-improve-sleepquality-idUSKBN1E12DK.

Photography Credits

Key: ph = photographer, a = above,
b = below, l = left, r = right.

p. 2 © Shutterstock.com/Mitch Johanson

p. 7 © CICO Books, ph. Peter Moore

p. 8 © Ryland Peters and Small, ph. Earl Carter

p. 11 © Ryland Peters and Small, ph. Debi Treloar

p. 12 © Ryland Peters and Small, ph. Chris Everard

p. 19 © Ryland Peters and Small, ph. Steve Painter

p. 22 © CICO Books, ph. David Merewether

p. 25 © Ryland Peters and Small, ph. Debi Treloar

p. 27 © Ryland Peters and Small, ph. Earl Carter

p. 28 © CICO Books, ph. Dylan Drummond

p. 31 © CICO Books, ph. Mark Scott

p. 37 © CICO Books, ph. Dylan Drummond

p. 39 © Ryland Peters and Small, ph. Chris Tubbs

p. 40 © Ryland Peters and Small, ph. Chris Tubbs

p. 41 © CICO Books, ph. Helen Cathcart

p. 45 © Shutterstock.com/Mitch Johanson

p. 47 © CICO Books, ph. Edina van der Wyck

p. 49 © Ryland Peters and Small, ph. Steve Painter

p. 52 © CICO Books, ph. Helen Cathcart

p. 55 © Shutterstock.com/Riccardo Arata

p. 57 © Shutterstock.com/jeff speigner

p. 61a © Shutterstock.com/P A

p. 61b © Shutterstock.com/images72

p. 65 © CICO Books, ph. Helen Cathcart

p. 67 © Ryland Peters and Small, ph. Caroline Hughes

p. 68 © Ryland Peters and Small, ph. Clare Winfield

p. 69 © Ryland Peters and Small, ph. Tara Fisher

p. 71 © Shutterstock.com/barmalini

p. 73 © Shutterstock.com/Vasin Lee

p. 74 © CICO Books, ph. David Merewether